THE ESSENTIAL FOOD LISTS FOR THE GLYCEMIC LOAD DIET

DISCOVER THE BEST AND WORST FOODS FOR WEIGHT LOSS AND DIABETES — WITH THE GI & GL VALUES OF OVER 2000 FOODS

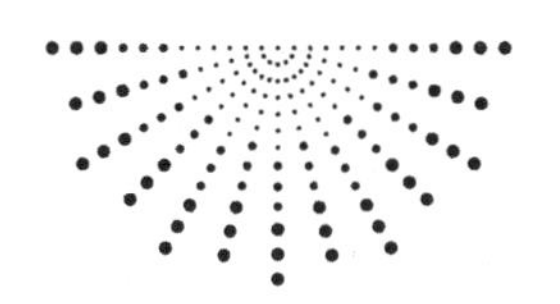

DR. H. MAHER

ISBN: 9798848165388

Medical Disclaimer: Because each individual is different and has particular dietary needs or restrictions, the dieting and nutritional information provided in this book does not constitute professional advice and is not a substitute for expert medical advice. Individuals should always check with a doctor before undertaking "a dieting, weight loss, or exercise regimen and should continue only under a doctor's supervision. While we provide the advice and information in this book in the hopes of helping individuals improve their overall health, multiple factors influence a person's results, and individual results may vary. When a doctor's advice to a particular individual conflicts with advice provided in this book, that individual should always follow the doctor's advice. Patients should not stop taking any of their medications without the consultation of their physician.

❀ Created with Vellum

CONTENTS

INTRODUCTION

"What can I eat and how much?" is one of the main questions asked by people who want to lose weight or those who want to prevent or delay type 2 diabetes—and the aim of this book is to help answer that question and provide dieters and people with diabetes or at risk for type 2 diabetes with powerful tools.

Adhering to the glycemic load diet is more than selecting foods you eat, restricting your carbohydrate intake, and avoiding foods that cause high blood sugar spikes; it's also about sticking to the proper lifestyle that promotes a healthy weight, better diabetes management, healthier life, and well-being. Thus, you have to focus simultaneously on your diet and lifestyle to reap all benefits of the glycemic load diet in terms of weight loss, weight maintenance, and diabetes management.

You can only focus on diet and keep your habits, but you'll not experience optimum health, lose weight, reach a healthy weight, or prevent and control diabetes. The two significant areas in which change is highly advised are physical activity and sleeping habits. Practicing regular physical activity will drive many beneficial effects in improving blood sugar control and insulin sensitivity. It will also help you improve your overall health. Sleeping well helps your body and brain function correctly, boost your immune system, improve your mental health, and can improve your diabetes management and prevent, or delay, diabetes complications. By committing to these easy and positive changes, you will expect to achieve a healthy weight, better blood glucose control, positive health outcomes, and prevent diabetes complications.

THE BENEFITS OF THE LOW GLYCEMIC LOAD DIET

Lowering your insulin levels is one of the secrets to better glycemic control and management, lasting weight loss, and improved health conditions. High insulin levels caused by eating high glycemic load foods are harmful and promote long-term high blood fat, high blood glucose, high blood pressure, and increase the risk of a heart attack. Because of this, following the low glycemic load diet is beneficial in controlling your blood sugar level, driving weight loss in the mid and long-term, preventing diabetes, PCOS, and heart disease, and improving your overall health.

Unlike other popular low-carbohydrates, high protein diets, eating a low glycemic load diet has been scientifically proven to help people:

- lose weight and maintain a healthy weight
- control blood sugar and lower insulin release
- reduce the risk of developing type 2 diabetes
- improve women's gestational diabetes management and reduce adverse pregnancy outcomes
- prevent diabetes complications
- achieve and maintain a healthy weight

- reduce PCOS symptoms
- maintain a healthy condition
- reduce the risk of developing metabolic syndrome significantly
- prevent heart attack and stroke

Conversely, consuming high glycemic load foods may be harmful to your health and causes high spikes in your blood sugar compared to low glycemic load foods.

High glycemic load food consumption has also been associated with an increased risk of diabetes complications, a higher risk of obesity, insulin resistance, fatty liver, metabolic syndrome, and an elevated risk of chronic disease.

Low-glycemic load Diet is Better for Your Body

Carbohydrates found in natural foods, such as legumes, fruits, vegetables, meats, fish, and grains, tend to be more complex and harder to digest and generally have low glycemic index values. Eating such foods will lead to smooth increases and falls in your blood glucose levels, which help you improve your overall health, prevent obesity, help diabetes control, and prevent diabetes complications.

Low-glycemic load diet leads to hunger-reduction

Leptin, referred to as the starvation or "hunger hormone," is a hormone produced by fat tissues and is released into your bloodstream. It plays an essential role in weight regulation by reducing a person's appetite.

Eating low glycemic load foods translates to eating foods that lower the insulin response and increase circulating leptin levels inducing a post-meal condition favorable for reduced food consumption due to a lower person's appetite. This may be very beneficial in such situations:

- type 2 diabetes management
- obesity control
- weight loss
- weight maintenance management
- insulin resistance

When you eat the right foods, you will notice that your appetite is under control due to the leptin effect. Your insulin levels will also be more stabilized, and your sugar levels will rise and falls smoothly.

Low-glycemic load diet and Insulin Resistance Reversal

Insulin resistance is a serious and silent health condition that occurs when cells in your muscles, liver, and body fat start ignoring the signal that the insulin hormone is sending out to transfer sugar out of the bloodstream and put it into your body cells. As insulin resistance develops, the body reacts by producing more and more insulin to lower blood sugar.

Over time, the β cells in the pancreas working hard to make a higher supply of insulin can no longer provide more and more insulin. Your blood sugar then reflects the pancreas' failure to maintain the level in the healthy range, and your blood sugar rises, showing prediabetes or, at worst, diabetes type 2.

Insulin resistance is silent and presents no symptoms in the first stage of its development. The symptoms appear later when the condition worsens, and the pancreas cannot produce enough insulin to keep your blood sugar within the normal range. When this occurs, the symptoms may be severe including, metabolic syndrome, polycystic ovary syndrome (PCOS), and various types of diabetes.

Fortunately, it is possible to reduce the effects of insulin resistance and boost your insulin sensitivity by following a low-glycemic index diet.

PART I
THE GLYCEMIC LOAD DIET EXPLAINED

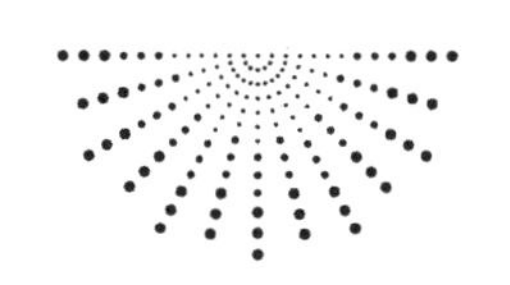

1

FOOD, WEIGHT LOSS AND DIABETES

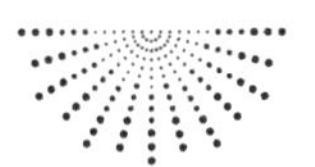

Eating to lower blood sugar spikes is not a one-size-fits-all approach. Different people, even twins, may respond to the same foods very differently. However, following the glycemic load dietary pattern will ensure you get the most of its beneficial effects. People who adhere to this diet more closely have consistently lower levels of blood sugar levels, lower blood pressure, increased LDL cholesterol, reduced HDL cholesterol, and reduced triglycerides than those following other diets. It is considered healthier than modern fad diets (e.g., keto diet, low-carb, high-fat diets) because it is centered around eating low glycemic, unprocessed, or minimally processed foods and avoiding high glycemic foods and pro-inflammatory agents.

- **Diet, Weight Loss, and Diabetes**

For years, hundreds of diets have been created with a lot of promises in terms of weight loss, inflammation reduction, and diabetes reversal. Low-fat diets, and low carb high fats diets were thought to be the best approaches to losing weight, controlling diabetes, and achieving a healthy weight. However, a growing and strong body of evidence shows that these diets often don't work:

- low-fat diets have the tendency to replace fat with easily digested carbohydrates.
- low-carb high-fat diets overlook the importance of carbohydrates and often replace carbohydrates with highly processed fat-containing foods.
- fad diets often overlook the body's fundamental need for a balanced diet

The best diets that work, restrict calories to some extent, supply sufficient and high-quality nutrients, banish bad foods, and balance hormones that help lower your blood sugar, improve your glycemic control, and regulate your weight. Diets do this in three main ways:

1. getting you to eat sufficient good foods and/or banish bad ones
2. getting you aware of foods and nutrients you should include in your diet to achieve weight loss, better diabetes control, and prevent complications.
3. changing some of your bad eating habits and the ways you consider highly processed foods and refined carbohydrates

The best diet for losing weight and/or diabetes control is one that is good for all body parts, from your brain to your heart to your pancreas. It is also a diet you can embrace and live with for a long time. In other words, a powerful diet rooted in nature that offers a flexible eating pattern, provides healthy choices, banishes unhealthy foods, and doesn't require an extensive (and probably expensive) shopping list or supplements.

A healthy balanced diet with sufficient and right nutritional elements is critical for battling diabetes, weight gain, and obesity. Both nutritional deficiency and excess are tied with diseases and poor health conditions. Nutritional excess, particularly in highly-processed foods, refined carbohydrates, saturated fats, trans-fatty acids, sugar-sweetened foods, and sodium, can result in severe chronic inflammatory illnesses such as autoimmune disease, cardiovascular disease, bone disorders, diabetes as well as obesity. In contrast, nutritional deficiencies can lead to impairments of body function, fatigue, and conditions associated with vitamin and mineral deficiencies.

One diet that allows that is a Low glycemic load type diet. Such a diet —and its many variations—usually include:

- several servings of plant foods (e.g., vegetables, fruits) a day
- whole and minimally processed foods
- daily serving of seeds and nuts
- healthy fats and oils high in omega-3 fatty acids (canola, cod liver oil, fatty fish, flaxseed oil, Walnut oil, sunflower oil, etc.)
- lean protein mainly from fish, poultry, and nuts
- limited amounts of red meat
- limited amounts of sodium
- very limited quantities of refined carbohydrates (e.g., white flour, white, rice, white sugar, brown sugar, honey, corn syrup)
- limited alcoholic drinks
- NO high glycemic load foods
- NO trans fats
- NO highly processed foods

- **Dietary carbohydrates and diabetes**

Increased intake of carbohydrates-containing foods with a higher glycemic index is found to cause a high spike in blood sugar and insulin release, making it harder to lose weight, control diabetes, and increase the risk of developing diabetes for healthy people. Conversely, eating carbohydrates-containing foods with a low glycemic load is associated with positive health outcomes and weight loss.

In addition, many studies have established that the quality of carbohydrates has a significant impact on inflammation, weight gain, insulin resistance, and the occurrence of diabetes complications. Low-quality carbohydrates such as highly processed foods and refined carbs are associated with increased inflammation, both acute and chronic, impaired immune system responses, poor blood glucose control, and increased risk of diabetes complications. Conversely, high-quality foods such as whole foods or minimally processed food with low glycemic load food are linked with lasting weight loss and better health outcomes, including improved control of blood glucose, and reduced acute and chronic inflammation.

- **Dietary fats and diabetes**

Another important nutrient you should consider as part of a glycemic load diet is fat. Eating a sufficient amount of good fat is essential whether you are managing diabetes or aiming to achieve a healthy weight.

However, fats are higher in calories per gram compared to proteins or carbohydrates. A gram of dietary fat has nearly 9 calories, while a gram of carbohydrate has roughly 4 calories or protein has about 4 calories. Thus, you should be aware of serving sizes when eating fats.

Several studies have established that replacing trans fats and saturated fats with unsaturated fats (monounsaturated and polyunsaturated) reduces the risk of cardiovascular diseases in high-risk populations, including individuals with diabetes.

In addition, studies also found that replacing trans fats and saturated fat intake with low glycemic carbohydrates (e.g., whole grains, fiber-rich fruits, fiber-rich vegetables, beans) results in cardiovascular benefits without altering the blood glucose control.

On the other side, a growing body of evidence has revealed how dietary fat intake affects the inflammatory status and focused on the gut microbiome as an important factor explaining the increase of inflammation biomarkers and fat intake. Trans fats are tied with various adverse health effects, worsen inflammation, and trigger some diabetes complications. The consumption of high amounts of saturated fats increases the LDL cholesterol (bad form) promotes and aggravates inflammation.

The American Diabetes Association recommends swapping saturated and trans fats in your diet with the healthiest alternatives such as monounsaturated and polyunsaturated fats.

2

THE GLYCEMIC LOAD DIET FOR WEIGHT LOSS OR DIABETES CONTROL

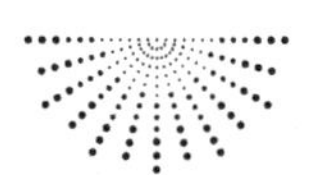

If you search for low-glycemic diets online, you'll find a lot of promising weight-loss miracles along without any evidence-based science or related research. Suppose you decide to go further and try to implement such methods. In that case, you will be sure to run into flaws and inconsistencies because the GL diet, unlike many other diets, didn't provide formal guidelines nor provide optimal daily foods intake as many claims.

Keeping in mind that the glycemic load diet is instead an eating plan or a lifestyle will increase your awareness of achieving a lasting weight loss or maintaining a healthy condition by eating according to the glycemic index.

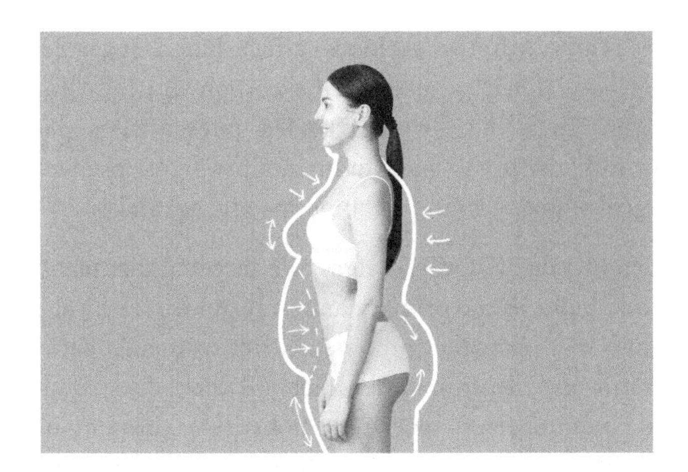

Fortunately, the science behind weight loss is today better developed, especially the link between hormones and weight gain and obesity. Therefore, if you want to lose weight, you have to understand how some specific hormones are involved in the weight gain process and how to make them work for you by eating good carbohydrates (low-GI foods).

THE GLYCEMIC INDEX DIET

The glycemic index (GI) was initially developed in the early 1980s to scientifically determine how different foods containing carbohydrates — vegetables, legumes, fruits, processed foods, and dairy products — affect blood sugar levels. Since that initial research led by Dr. Jenkins took place more than 35 years ago, many scientists have come to identify the opportunity that the glycemic index (GI) can be a powerful tool for maintaining weight, improving the effectiveness of weight-loss diets, and managing diabetes.

The glycemic index isn't formally a diet in the sense that you have to conform to strict rules, follow particular meal plans or eliminate some foods from your daily meals. Instead, it's a scientific method of identifying how carbohydrates in foods affect blood sugar levels and measuring how slowly or quickly the carbohydrates in foods raise blood sugar. Thus, the Glycemic Index referential is particularly important to know if you want to maintain weight, lose weight, take more control of diabetes, and fix some specific health issues.

The "glycemic index (GI) diet" refers to a targeted diet plan that uses the glycemic index as the primary and only guides for meal planning. Unlike other diet plans that provide a strict recommendation with a specific ratio, the glycemic index diet (GI diet) doesn't specify the optimal daily number of calories, carbohydrates, protein, or fats for weight maintenance or weight loss. Instead, it provides an effective eating plan with more flexibility and sustainable results in weight loss, weight management, and diabetes control.

UNDERSTANDING GI VALUES

Glycemic index (GI) values are divided into three categories:

- Low GI: This category comprises foods that have their GI value below 55
- Medium GI: This category comprises foods that have their GI value in the range 56 to 69
- High GI: In general, this category must be avoided because foods cause high spikes in the blood sugar level. Their GI value are equal or higher to 70

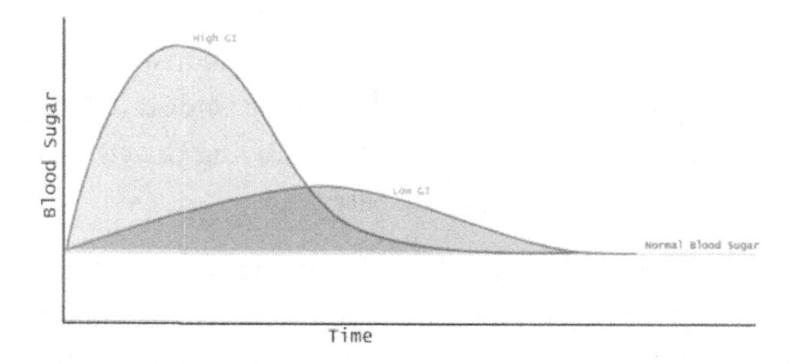

Comparing the GI values may help guide your food choices. For example, muesli has a GI value of approximately 86. A vegetable and fruit smoothie drink has a GI value of 55.

HOW DOES GLYCEMIC INDEX (GI) DIET WORK?

Eating according to the Glycemic Index Diet looks simple because all you need to know is where different foods fall on the 0 to 100 glycemic index (GI).

- You fill up on low GI foods (GI value: 55 and under)
- Eat smaller amounts of medium GI foods (GI value:56 to 69)
- And mostly avoid high GI foods (GI value: 70 and up)

Besides referring to the glycemic index lists as needed, there is no difficult weighing or measuring and no need to track your calorie intake. However, you will have to concoct your eating plan and menus yourself.

HOW IS GLYCEMIC INDEX MEASURED?

Glycemic Index values of foods are measured using valid and proven scientific methods and cannot be guessed just by looking at the composition of specific food or the nutrition facts on food packaging.

Thus, the GI calculation Follows the international standard method and provides values that are commonly accepted. The Glycemic Index value of food is calculated by feeding over ten healthy people a portion of the food object of the study and containing fifty grams of digestible carbohydrate and then measuring the effect for each participant on his blood glucose levels (blood glucose response) over the next two hours.

The second part of the process consists of giving the same participants an equal carbohydrate portion of the glucose (used as the reference food) and measuring their blood glucose response over the next two hours.

The Glycemic Index value for the food is then calculated for each participant by using a simple formula (dividing the blood glucose response for the food by their blood glucose response for the glucose (reference food)). The final value of the Glycemic Index for the food is the average Glycemic Index value for the participants (over 10).

Carbohydrates with a low GI value (55 or less) are more slowly digested, absorbed, and metabolized and induce a smaller and slower rise in blood glucose and, therefore, usually, insulin levels.

Low glycemic diets or foods are associated with a reduced risk of chronic disease. Foods that have a low glycemic index are known for their ability to release glucose in the blood slowly and regularly. Conversely, Foods that have a high glycemic index are known for their property to release glucose rapidly. Researches suggest that foods with a low glycemic index (LGI foods) are ideal for weight loss diets and foster lasting weight loss, in addition to their positive effect on the pancreas (insulin release), eyes, and kidney.

THE GLYCEMIC LOAD CONCEPT

Basing your food choices only on the GI means that you're focusing on only one aspect of the food and ignoring other important aspects, such as the quality and quantity of the carbohydrates in the foods. Here comes the importance of the glycemic load, which combines the two criteria and provides, when available, an additional tool for better weight loss control and effective diabetes management.

The glycemic Load was developed later by Harvard researchers to provide a more useful tool that allows to track of both carbohydrates quality and quantity. The glycemic load of a specific food—computed as the product of that food's glycemic index value and its net carbohydrates content —has direct physiologic significance in that each unit of GL corresponds to the glycemic effect of ingesting 1 g of glucose. Typical low-glycemic diets contain from 50–150 GL units per day. **For optimal health outcomes, it is highly recommended to keep your daily glycemic load (GL) under 100. This will help achieve a healthy weight, and keep your A1C level in the normal range. If you have diabetes, you can eat up to 50 grams of sugar from all sources per day (in a 2,000-calorie diet). This means that you should target a GL of 50.**

The Glycemic Load (GL) is computed using the following formula:

Glycemic Load (GL) = GI x Net Carbohydrates (grams) content per portion ÷ 100

Where net carbohydrate = total carbohydrates - dietary fiber

One unit of GL corresponds to the glycemic effect of ingesting 1 g of glucose. Typical low glycemic load diets contain from 80–150 GL units per day.

As shown in the formula, the GL of a food is a product of 2 factors: the GI of the food and the net carb in food for a given serving size. And thus, to increase or decrease GL you have to act primarily on the serving size. Therefore, low GL food can be obtained by reducing the serving size.

GLYCEMIC LOAD RANGES

Like the glycemic index, the glycemic load (GL) of a food can be classified as:

- **Low:** 10 or less

- **Medium:** 11 – 19
- **High:** 20 or more

For a standard serving size of food, glycemic load (GL) is considered high with GL greater or equal to 20, medium with GL in the range of 11-19, and low with GL less or equal to 10. The Daily GL is the sum of the GL values for all foods consumed during the day.

Because there is a gap in the GL ranges, a food with a glycemic load (GL) of 10.1 is considered a medium GL. A food with a glycemic load (GL) of 19.1 is considered a High GL.

Eating frequently many high glycemic load foods is associated with an increased risk for type 2 diabetes, cardiovascular disease, overweight, and obesity. Conversely, eating low glycemic foods has been shown to help control type 2 diabetes, improve blood markers and improve weight loss.

THE GLYCEMIC LOAD AND PORTION SIZES

Because the Glycemic Load of food is a function of the food's glycemic index and net carb content of the considered portion of the food, it is evident that the estimated GL value will change if you change the serving size. To illustrate this observation, let's consider watermelon fruit.

- Watermelon fruit has a glycemic index of 72 (high)
- One cup of diced watermelon (152 grams) contains about 11.5 grams of total carbs and 0.5 grams of fiber, implying that watermelon has roughly 11 grams of net carbs.

The glycemic load of watermelon for one-cup serving size (152 grams) equals 7.92. (Low GL)

The glycemic load of watermelon for a much large serving (190 grams) equals 9.90. (Low GL)

The glycemic load of watermelon for a much large serving (240 grams) equals 12.50. (Medium GL)

Now, let's consider sweet potato.

- Sweet Potato Casserole Or Mashed has a high glycemic index: GI= 66 (medium)
- One cup of Sweet Potato Casserole Or Mashed (250 grams) contains about 53.75 grams of net carbs.

The glycemic load of Sweet Potato Casserole Or Mashed for a One-cup (250-grams) serving size equals 25.7 (High GL)

The glycemic load of Sweet Potato Casserole Or Mashed for a ⅔ cup (166-grams) serving size equals 16.5 (Medium GL)

The glycemic load of Sweet Potato Casserole Or Mashed for a ⅓ cup (83-grams) serving size equals 8.6 (Low GL)

The glycemic load (GL) of a meal is obtained by adding the glycemic loads of all foods consumed.

FACTORS AFFECTING A FOOD'S GLYCEMIC LOAD

Many factors affect the glycemic load of food. These factors include:

Food Processing Methods: Food processing has been practiced for centuries in form of cooking, dehydrating, fermenting, ultraviolet radiation, and salt preservation. However, modern food processing methods are more sophisticated and complex, and alter considerably foods, by adding many ingredients including trans fats, high-fructose corn syrup, salts, artificial sweeteners, flavors, colors, and other chemical additives. The U.S. Department of Agriculture (USDA) defines processed food as one that has undergone any procedure that alters it from its natural state. Highly Processed foods tend to have a higher glycemic index and glycemic load because they contain added sugar and are so refined that you digest them more easily than minimally processed alternatives.

Ripeness: when fruits or vegetables ripen, their nutritional compositions change significantly. Sugar content increases as the fruit or starchy vegetables ripen as part of the ripening process. The starch in fruits or vegetables is transformed into sugars, and the proportion of simple sugar rises to roughly 20%. Therefore ripe and over-ripe foods have generally higher glycemic index and glycemic load than unripe ones.

Physical form: Complex carbohydrates are formed by sugar molecules that are linked together in complex and long chains. Complex carbs are digested slowly and did not cause high spikes in your blood sugar. Conversely, simple or refined carbohydrates are transformed quickly by the body and induce powerful spikes in blood sugar. Therefore, refined and simple carbohydrates-containing foods have generally higher glycemic index and glycemic load than complex carbs.

GLYCEMIC LOAD OF A MIXED MEAL

The use of GL values of individual foods to estimate the average GL value of a meal may be appropriate. You may add the GL values of foods to estimate the glycemic load of a meal.

Should people with diabetes eat a Glycemic Load diet?

Whereas the glycemic index is a good tool for making good food choices, the glycemic load, goes beyond and helps to work out how different portions sizes of different foods compare with each other and thus help you eat the right serving sizes that would not cause high spikes in your blood sugar.

WILL GLYCEMIC LOAD DIET HELP YOU LOSE WEIGHT?

Low-glycemic diets demonstrate short-term and mid-term weight loss much more than other diets show. Eating low glycemic load foods, and keeping your daily glycemic load under 100 is the key to weight loss and hormonal balance. A 2012 study published in the Journal of "The American Medical Association" found low glycemic diets to be best and superior at maintaining weight loss when compared to very low carbohydrates diets (like the ketogenic or keto diet) and low-fat diets. The findings support the low glycemic diet's assumption that "a calorie is not a calorie" and that "different kinds of food will affect us in different ways, despite having the same calories' number". Another paper published in "The American Journal of Clinical Nutrition" in 2014 supports low Glycemic and calorie-restricted diets as more effective than high Glycemic Index and low-fat diets for weight management and weight loss.

LIMITATIONS OF THE CONCEPT

The glycemic index and glycemic load are great tools, but they do have a few limitations that you need to know:

- The lists of GI are quite limited. G.I. testing is new, and the process is expensive, time and resource-consuming.
- The glycemic index depends on some external intervention like cooking. Al Dente Pasta is known to have a Lower Glycemic Index
- The testing results may vary. Researchers rely on the observation of tests involving participants' metabolism to measure glycemic index as explained in the previous section. This explains why GI may vary among studies.

Despite these limitations, the glycemic load is a very useful tool that will help you achieve your goals in terms of weight loss, health, and disease prevention.

3
THE GLYCEMIC LOAD LIFESTYLE FOR BETTER DIABETES MANAGEMENT

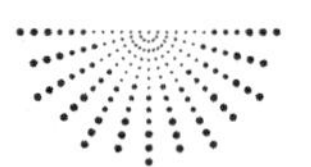

Adhering to the glycemic load for diabetes is more than selecting foods you eat, restricting your daily GL, and avoiding high glycemic index foods; it's also about sticking to the proper lifestyle that promotes better diabetes management, healthier life, and well-being. Thus, you have to focus simultaneously on your diet and lifestyle to reap all benefits of the glycemic load for diabetes and improve your blood sugar control and heart health.

You can only focus on diet and keep your habits, but you'll not experience optimum health and win your battle against diabetes. The two significant areas in which change is highly advised are physical activity and sleeping habits. Practicing regular physical activity will drive many beneficial effects in improving blood sugar control and insulin sensitivity. It will also help you prevent, delay, and reduce morbidities and complications associated with diabetes Mellitus. Sleeping well helps your body and brain function correctly, boost your immune system, improve your mental health, and can improve your diabetes management and prevent, or delay, diabetes complications. By committing to these easy and positive changes, you will expect to achieve better blood glucose control, positive health outcomes, and prevent diabetes complications.

Based on the best and latest science of how and what to eat, the diabetes glycemic load lifestyle is meant to be your global road map for managing diabetes, which is the key to preventing, reducing, or delaying complications. You are advised to use "ABCDEs of diabetes" as a way to manage your new diabetes glycemic index lifestyle:

- A- A stands for A1C, or HbA1c test, which assesses your blood glucose control over the past two to three months. So, get a regular A1C (HbA1c) test to measure your average blood glucose and target to stay under 7% as much as possible.
- B- B refers to blood pressure. Nearly 50% of people with type 2 diabetes suffer from hypertension. Try to keep your blood pressure below 130/80 mm Hg (or 140/90 mm Hg in some cases).
- C- C refers to cholesterol. Total blood cholesterol, HDL cholesterol (good), LDL cholesterol (bad), and triglycerides levels should be monitored. Your doctor will use the information and, if needed, develop a strategy to reduce your risks.
- D- D refers to diet. It refers to adhering to the glycemic load diet for diabetes and, if indicated, drug therapy. Your doctor may prescribe medicines that may help you lower your blood glucose, blood pressure (if applicable), cholesterol, and triglyceride levels (if applicable).
- E- E refers to exercice. You should practice regular physical activities for at least 150 minutes per week (e.g., 30 minutes, 6 days a week).

PART II
UNDERSTANDING HORMONES THAT CONTROL YOUR WEIGHT

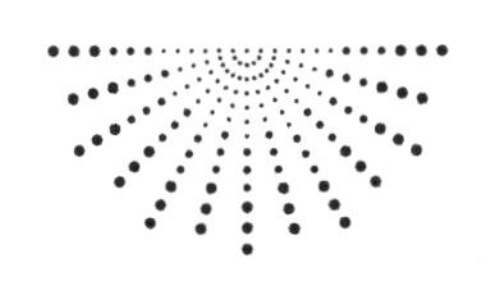

4
THE INSULIN HORMONE

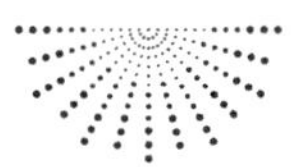

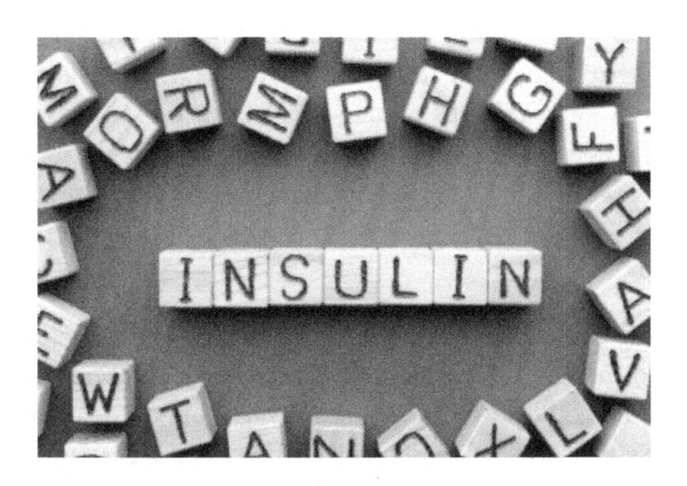

Insulin is an essential hormone involved in many metabolic processes affecting weight loss and weight gain mechanisms. Made by the pancreas, insulin regulates the absorption of sugar by body cells and maintains the sugar level present in the blood at a healthy level. When you eat, food moves through your esophagus into your stomach and intestines to be broken down into micronutrients absorbed and transported by your bloodstream. The pancreas produces and releases insulin and releases it into the bloodstream when we eat to allow body cells, including muscles and other cells, to absorb and transform sugar (glucose) into energy throughout the body.

Insulin also signals to the liver, muscle, and adipocytes (fat cells) to store the excess glucose for further use. Extra sugar is stored in 3 ways:

- In muscle tissues as glycogen.
- In the liver as glycogen.
- In adipose tissue (fat reserves of the body) as triglycerides which are fat molecules that store energy

WEIGHT GAIN AND INSULIN

In theory, it's impossible to gain weight if you eat no carbohydrates because the pancreas will not release insulin, the only polypeptide hormone that induces fat storage into adipose tissue. And thus, you can not have any more fat stored in your body. So, if you want to lose weight, it's essential that rises and falls in blood sugar must be as smooth as possible. The longer the digestion of carbohydrates takes, the better it is. And here came the importance of the glycemic index concept.

Remember that eating high glycemic index food cause a rapid rise in insulin hormone levels in the blood, translating to excess fat in the body. Insulin is the hormone that sends sugar out of the bloodstream into the tissue cells for use as energy. When extra sugar resides in the blood, insulin hormone levels stay high, and insulin signals to the body to store excess calories in the form of fat. Thus, High insulin hormone levels imply you'll have more body fat, while low insulin hormone levels mean you'll have less body fat.

INSULIN RESISTANCE

Insulin resistance is a serious and silent health condition that occurs when cells in your muscles, liver, and body fat start ignoring the signals that insulin is sending to move glucose out of the bloodstream and put it into your body cells. As insulin resistance develops, the body reacts by producing more and more insulin to lower blood sugar.

Insulin resistance is silent and presents no symptoms in the first stage of its development. The symptoms appear later when the condition worsens, and the pancreas cannot produce enough insulin to maintain healthy levels of blood sugar. When this occurs, the symptoms may be severe including, metabolic syndrome, polycystic ovary syndrome (PCOS), and various types of diabetes.

Fortunately, it is possible to reduce the effects of insulin resistance and boost your insulin sensitivity by following a low-glycemic load diet.

Thus, for many of you, adhering to the low-glycemic load diet goes beyond weight-loss management and target the management of particular health condition sensitive to such kind of diet and particularly those related to insulin resistance like:

- Excessive hunger
- Lethargy or tiredness
- Difficulty concentrating
- Brain fog
- Waist weight gain
- High blood pressure

5

THE CORTISOL HORMONE

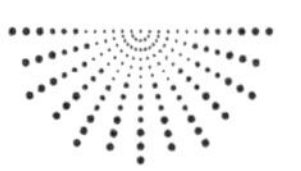

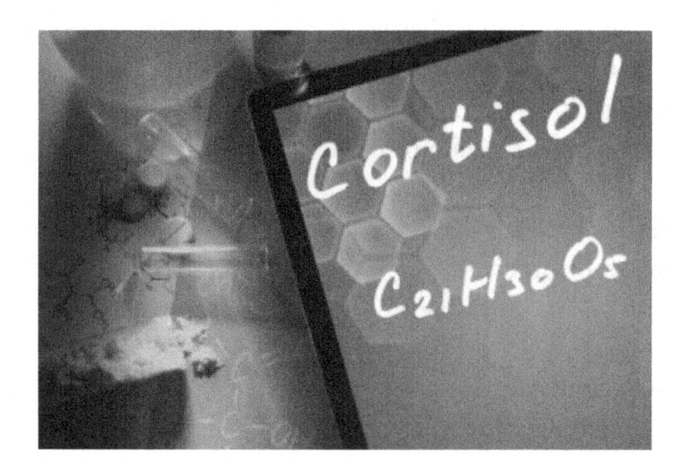

Cortisol is a steroid hormone made and released by the two adrenal glands when the body faces stressful situations. The hypothalamus, via the pituitary gland, sends a chemical signal to the adrenal glands to produce and release adrenaline and cortisol.

Cortisol is naturally released every day in small and regular quantities. However, like adrenaline, cortisol can also be secreted and released in reaction to physical and emotional stress and triggers the body's fight-or-flight response.

These two stress hormones work simultaneously: adrenaline significantly increases strength, performance, and awareness and increases metabolism. It also lets fat cells release additional energy. Cortisol helps the body make glucose from proteins and quickly increases the body's energy in times of stress.

However, cortisol is also involved in a variety of essential functions for your health. Most of the body cells have cortisol receptors to use this steroid hormone for a variety of critical functions, including:

- blood sugar regulation
- metabolism regulation
- inflammation reduction
- memory formulation

Cortisol is important for your health, but an excess of cortisol can harm your body and induce various undesired symptoms.

WHAT CAUSE HIGH CORTISOL LEVELS?

Several things can cause a high cortisol level, known as Cushing syndrome. This health condition results from your body secreting and releasing too much cortisol.

Cushing syndrome causes many undesired symptoms,

including:

- obesity
- weight gain
- fatty deposits, especially in the face, midsection, and between the shoulders
- purple stretch marks on the arms, breasts, thighs, and abdomen

- thinning skin
- slow-healing injuries

Being under stress induces a constant state of excess cortisol production. And, as seen above, this cortisol drives excess glucose production in a non-fight-or-flight situation. This excess glucose is converted into fat and stored by the body.

Thus, high cortisol levels increase the risk of obesity highly, induce abdominal obesity, and increase fat storage.

Other factors that cause peaks in cortisol production are carbohydrates deprivation (in a low-carb diet, for example) and overconsumption of simple carbohydrates.

In both cases, when blood sugar levels fall, this induces a surge of stress hormones, including cortisol and adrenaline.

STRESS HORMONES AND THEIR ROLE IN THE BODY

Stress hormones are released in reply to body stressors. Hormonal responses of the woman's body to stress are essential, provided they occur less frequently. They may become damaging and unhealthy when they happen too often. Prolonged exposure to porn induces severe brain damage and presents evidence that porn is not a healthy stressor.

Stress is habitually accompanied by high energy demand. Consequently, a severe stress situation induces a fast glucose release into the blood, which provides the required energy to deal with the stressful situation.

The principal players in the stress mechanism are:

- The adreno-corticotropic hormone (ACTH),
- The glucocorticoids such as cortisol, adrenaline, and noradrenaline.

When this happens, blood glucose levels rise concurrently with heart rate and blood pressure.

So at its simplest, stress leads to increased blood glucose, high heart rate, and blood pressure, which induces an increased insulin release.

6

THE LEPTIN HORMONE

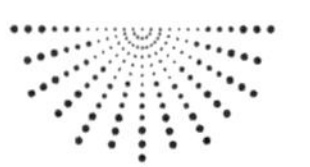

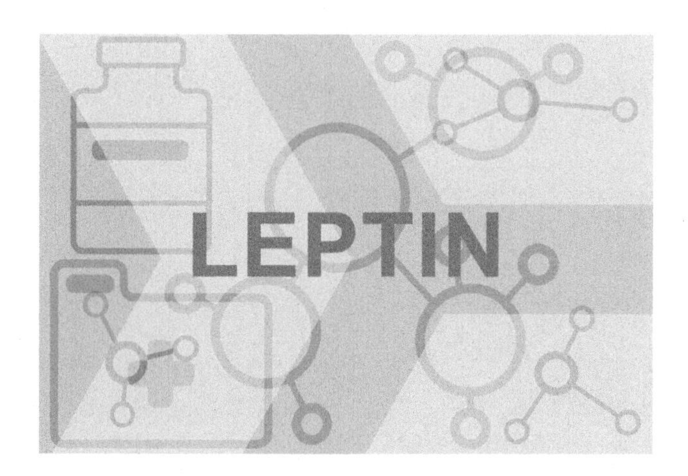

Leptin, referred to as the starvation or "hunger hormone, " is produced by fat tissues and secreted into our bloodstream. It plays an essential function in weight regulation by reducing a person's appetite.

The Leptin hormone was discovered in 1994 and has gained significant interest for its powerful role in weight regulation and obesity. Leptin communicates with specific centers of the brain to influence how the body manages its store of fat. It signals to the brain that the body has enough stored fat, inducing the body to burn calories from stored fat and reduce appetite.

Leptin plays the key regulator of body fat and signals the brain to burn stored fat. This powerful effect would usually prevent obesity, and overweight. Early research has seen leptin as the solution for obesity. A supplementation of leptin was thought to induce and sustain body fat burning, weight loss, and weight gain prevention. However, the clinical trials were inconclusive.

LEPTIN RESISTANCE

Because fat tissues produce leptin, it is released in the bloodstream proportionally to a person's weight. Leptin levels are high for people who are overweight or obese than for people having average weight.

However, research has shown that leptin's benefit in appetite-reducing is very low for obese people, suggesting that people with obesity aren't sensitive to the beneficial effect of leptin and have developed Leptin resistance.

Ongoing research focuses on leptin resistance in obese people, which stops the brain from acknowledging the leptin's signal. Some studies, however, suggest that obesity induces multiple cellular processes that attenuate or prevent leptin signaling, amplifying the extent of weight gain. Leptin Resistance may arise from poor leptin transport across the blood-brain barrier (BBB), alteration of the leptin receptor, and defect of leptin signaling...

WAYS TO IMPROVE LEPTIN RESISTANCE AND PROMOTE WEIGHT LOSS

Strong evidence shows that Leptin resistance can be drastically reduced by following these guidelines:

- Eat low-glycemic and medium-glycemic foods
- Avoid Ultra-processed food: the impact of Ultra-processed food is still under study, but many pieces of evidence suggest that these kinds of foods compromise the integrity of your gut, the normal functioning, and the production of gut hormones.
- Lower your triglycerides: Having high triglycerides levels in your bloodstream can prevent the transport of leptin to your brain.
- Eat healthy protein: Eating healthy proteins can improve leptin sensitivity.
- Eat healthy fats and keep your ratio of omega 6/ omega 3 inferior to 3.
- Avoid simple carbohydrates, and starches, and eat healthy carbohydrates (complex carbs, fiber).

7

THE GHRELIN HORMONE

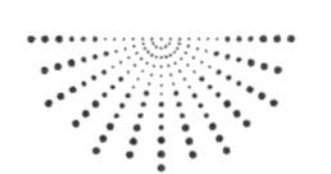

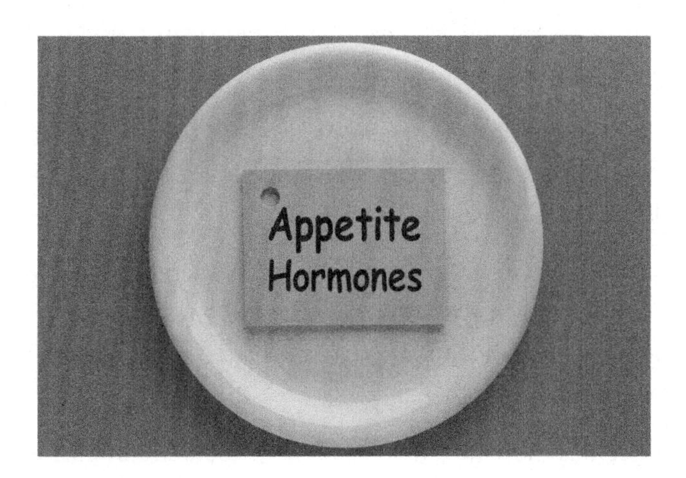

Ghrelin, known as the "hunger hormone," is an acyl-peptide responsible for stimulating hunger by sending a chemical signal to tell you when to eat. Ghrelin is made and released primarily by the stomach. The small intestine and pancreas also secrete smaller amounts of this hormone.

Ghrelin has various functions. It is known mainly as the hormone that triggers hunger by stimulating the appetite. It induces increases in food intake and promotes fat storage and weight gain.

These findings suggest that by controlling the level of gherkin and letting it down, we can reduce appetite and food intake.

An experiment administering ghrelin to people concluded that food intake was increased by 30% in this population.

HOW IS GHRELIN CONTROLLED?

Ghrelin levels are mainly regulated by food intake. Levels of ghrelin in the bloodstream rise typically before eating and when fasting in line with increased hunger.

Experimental studies demonstrated that Ghrelin levels are lower in obese or overweight individuals. Conversely, lean individuals have a high level of ghrelin.

Studies also found that some foods (low-GI foods) slow down the ghrelin released in the bloodstream and thus reduce the impact of hunger hormones.

Soluble and insoluble fibers inhibit ghrelin secretion, implying that eating complex carbohydrates (low-GI and medium-GI foods) will have a positive and substantial effect on reducing the production and release of ghrelin.

Glucose also has the same effect as dietary fibers in inhibiting Ghrelin secretion. However, as seen earlier, glucose, starches, and simple carbohydrates must be prohibited due to their impact on rising insulin release.

Recent studies demonstrated that, contrary to a common belief, proteins did not reduce the production or release of ghrelin.

8

THE PYY FAMILY

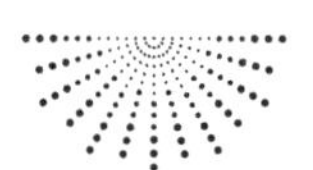

The gut hormone peptide PYY3–36 is a polypeptide hormone released from L-cells found in the large intestine and the intestinal mucosa of the ileum.

The hormone PYY is secreted and released proportionally to nutrient intake. The PYY levels become low in the fasting state but quickly increase in response to nutrient intake and remain high for several hours. The amount of the hormone PYY is also strongly influenced by the number of calories consumed, and the macronutrient and micronutrient composition of the eaten meal.

The primary role of the hormone PYY is to reduce appetite, which is the main psychological driver for eating. It also plays an important function in regulating the energy balance in the body.

Higher levels of PYY result in reduced appetite and may help in weight loss. Conversely, low levels of PYY induce strong feelings of hunger and cravings while predisposing fatty tissue retention.

PART III
UNDERSTANDING DIABETES AND INSULIN RESISTANCE

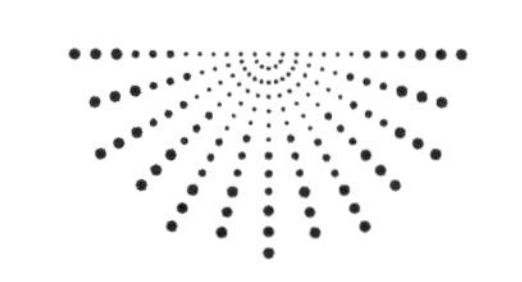

9
WHAT IS DIABETES?

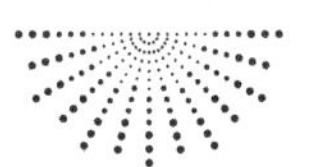

Diabetes is a chronic metabolic illness marked by unsuitable hyperglycemia due to a lack of insulin or insulin resistance. Its adverse health effects can seriously reduce life expectancy significantly by ten years. Several lifestyle factors and dietary habits affect the incidence of type 1 and type 2 diabetes, such as types and amounts of food ingested, weight gain, obesity, physical activity, watching TV or sedentary time, and sleep quality.

Diabetes mellitus refers to a chronic disease that influences how the body utilizes food for energy and is marked by abnormally high blood glucose levels. Insulin — the hormone made by the pancreas— allows glucose to get into body cells to provide energy. When blood sugar levels rise after eating, your pancreas releases a sufficient amount of insulin into the blood. Insulin then reduces blood sugar to keep it in the normal range. In people who have diabetes, the pancreas cannot perform this fundamental function, or the body's cells do not respond adequately to the produced insulin. The blood sugar level then increases, and sugar accumulates in the body and becomes toxic to the vital organs. Having a high glucose level in the blood can cause severe health problems. It can cause severe damage to the eyes, kidneys, heart, and nerves irreversibly.

Diabetes Mellitus is the most common chronic endocrine disorder caused mainly by inflammation according to recent high-quality research. There are three main types of diabetes:

- **1. Type 1 diabetes**

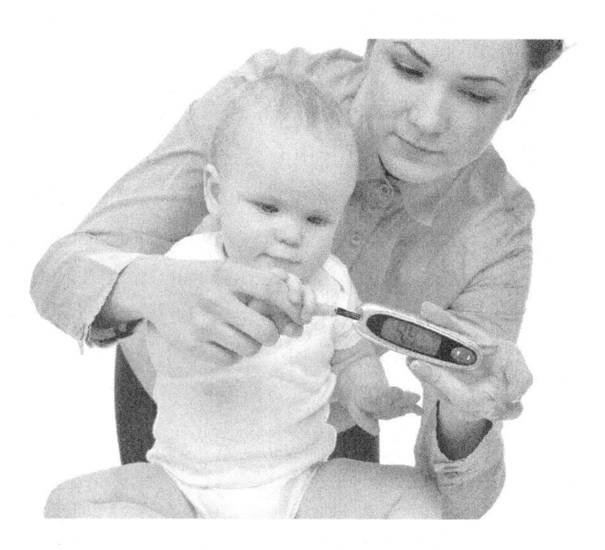

Type 1 diabetes mellitus (DM) is a chronic autoimmune disease characterized by the immune system's destruction of insulin-producing pancreatic *beta* cells. The body will no longer make insulin due to irreversible damage to the insulin-producing cells. Without insulin hormones, glucose can not get into the body's cells and the blood glucose increases above normal. People with type 1 must then inject daily insulin doses and follow a strict diet to stay alive and prevent the severe adverse effect. Type 1 diabetes generally appears in children and young adults but may occur at any age.

In 2016, the Food and Drug Administration approved the artificial pancreas to replace the manual blood glucose checking and the injection of insulin shots. These automated devices act like your real pancreas in controlling blood sugar and releasing insulin when the patient's blood sugar becomes too high. The artificial pancreas also releases a small flow of insulin continuously.

Symptoms of type 1 diabetes are serious and usually happen quickly, over a few days to weeks. Symptoms can include

- frequent thirst and urination
- increased hunger
- unexplained weight loss
- blurred vision
- frequent infections
- fatigue and tiredness

Unfortunately, type 1 DM is chronic immune-mediated and remains incurable. However, you can lower the risk of complications and improve its management by adhering to the glycemic load lifestyle.

- **2. Type 2 diabetes**

Prediabetes. Even if a person is not sick, he may suffer from prediabetes without knowing it. This term refers to an intermediate stage characterized by an abnormally higher blood glucose level than usual. That represents a warning signal that informs people with prediabetes diagnosis that they are at increased risk of type 2 diabetes mellitus if they don't take appropriate and urgent action, especially if they have other risk factors, including:

- overweight,
- obesity,

- sedentary lifestyle,
- high blood pressure.

In Type 2 diabetes, the mechanism is different from type 1 diabetes: insulin is normally secreted by the pancreas but with lower efficiency. Therefore, without sufficient insulin, the glucose stays in the blood. Type 2 diabetes is induced by several factors, including lifestyle factors, strict diets, overweight, obesity, Hyperthyroidism, and genes.

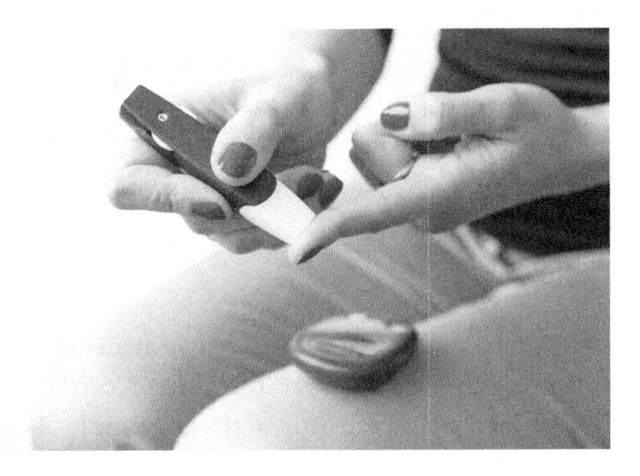

Type 2 diabetes (DM) can develop at any age. However, it's more common after the age of forty.

- **3. Gestational diabetes**

Gestational diabetes is the high blood sugar that develops during pregnancy in women who did not have diabetes before becoming pregnant. Gestational diabetes is more frequent in the second or third trimester but can occur at any time of pregnancy and usually disappears after giving birth.

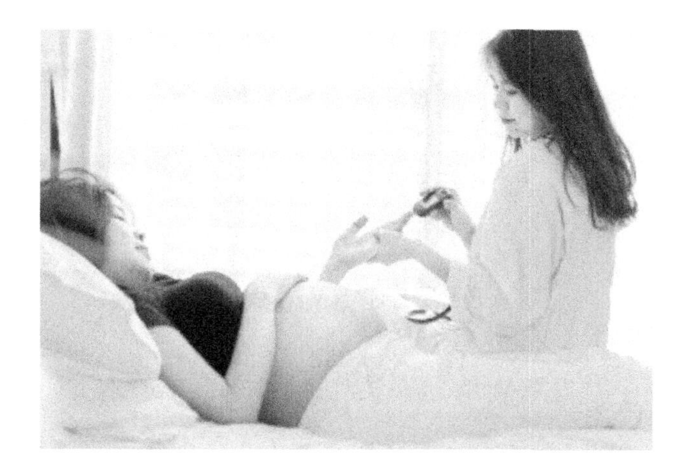

Women diagnosed with it are at higher risk of developing type 2 diabetes later in life, particularly for women with favoring factors (obesity, imbalanced diet, sedentary lifestyle, metabolic syndrome...).

10
DIABETES SYMPTOMS

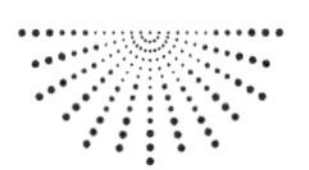

Symptoms of Type 1 Diabetes

If you have type 1 DM, you may experience, in addition to the common symptoms of diabetes, stomach pains, nausea, and vomiting. Type 1 diabetes symptoms can develop abruptly in just a few weeks and can be serious. Type 1 DM is an autoimmune illness that usually begins when you are children, a teen, or a young adult.

Symptoms of Type 2 Diabetes

Type 2 diabetes symptoms and signs develop slowly and can take years to develop. Some patients don't notice any symptoms at all until they got diagnosed. Type 2 diabetes generally begins when you are an adult, though more and more people are developing it at a young age due to excess consumption of sugar. Because symptoms are hard to identify or take longer to develop, it's crucial to be aware of the risk factors and visit your doctor accordingly. Risk factors include:

- overweight and obesity
- age 45 or older
- family history of diabetes

- high blood pressure condition
- heart disease or stroke condition
- polycystic ovary syndrome (PCOS)

Symptoms of Gestational Diabetes

Gestational diabetes typically doesn't induce any noticeable symptoms or signs. If you are pregnant, you may get tested for diabetes between 24 and 28 weeks of pregnancy.

Common Symptoms

Diabetes symptoms may vary depending on the level of blood sugar. Some people with prediabetes or type 2 diabetes may not experience frank symptoms at first. Conversely, with type 1 diabetes, symptoms come on quickly and severely.

Bellow a list of common symptoms and signs of type 1 and type 2 diabetes, and gestational diabetes:

- increased craving
- frequent urination
- excessive hunger
- weight loss
- ketones in urine
- fatigue and tiredness
- increased irritability
- blurred vision
- slow-healing wounds and cuts
- frequent infections

11
INSULIN RESISTANCE AND PREDIABETES

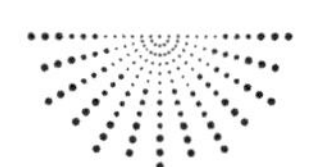

Insulin is a polypeptide hormone that controls and regulates the absorption of sugar by body cells and maintains the level of sugar present in the blood at a healthy level. This hormone is produced by the β cells of the pancreas. When you eat, food moves to your stomach and intestines to be broken down into micronutrients absorbed and transported by our bloodstream. The pancreas produces the insulin and releases it into the bloodstream when we eat to allow body cells, including muscles and other cells, to absorb and transform sugar (glucose) into energy throughout the body.

Insulin also signals to the liver, muscle, and adipocytes (fat cells) to store the excess glucose for further use. Extra sugar is stored in 3 ways:

- In muscle tissues as glycogen.
- In the liver as glycogen.
- In adipose tissue (fat reserves of the body) in the form of triglycerides which are fat molecules that store energy

INSULIN RESISTANCE

Insulin resistance is a serious and silent health condition that occurs when cells in your muscles, liver, and body fat start ignoring the signal that the insulin hormone is sending out to transfer sugar out of the bloodstream and put it into your body cells. As insulin resistance develops, the body reacts by producing more and more insulin to lower blood sugar.

Over time, the β cells in the pancreas working hard to make a higher supply of insulin can no longer provide more and more insulin. Your blood sugar may reflect the pancreas failure to maintain the level in the healthy range, and your blood sugar rises, showing pre-diabetes or, at worst, diabetes type 2.

Insulin resistance is silent and presents no symptoms in the first stage of its development. The symptoms appear later when the condition worsens, and the pancreas cannot produce enough insulin to keep your blood sugar within the normal range. When this occurs, the symptoms may be severe including, metabolic syndrome, polycystic ovary syndrome (PCOS), and various types of diabetes.

Fortunately, it is possible to reduce the effects of insulin resistance and boost your insulin sensitivity by following a low-glycemic load diet.

Thus, for many of you, following a low-glycemic diet goes beyond weight-loss management and target the management of particular health condition sensitive to such kind of diet and particularly those related to insulin resistance like:

- Excessive hunger
- Lethargy or tiredness
- Difficulty concentrating
- Brain fog
- Waist weight gain
- High blood pressure

Can insulin resistance be reduced or reversed?

Fortunately, It is possible to reduce the effects of insulin resistance and boost your insulin sensitivity by following some effective methods, including:

- Low glycemic load diet
- Low carbohydrate and high-fat diet
- Low-calorie diets
- Weight loss surgery
- Regular exercise in combination with healthy diets

These methods have a similar way of working. They all reduce the daily glucose intake drastically, lower the body's need for insulin, reduce insulin spikes in the bloodstream, promote weight loss and prevent weight gain.

12
DIABETES TESTS

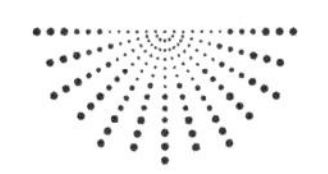

Diabetes, prediabetes, and gestational diabetes are diagnosed through blood tests which show if your blood sugar is too high. You'll need to get your blood glucose tested to determine if you have for sure prediabetes or type 1, type 2 diabetes, or gestational diabetes. Refrain yourself from self-diagnosing if you think you might have diabetes. Commercially available testing tools such as a blood glucose meter cannot diagnose diabetes. If you have symptoms of diabetes, you should see your doctor to get your blood sugar tested. Testing is quick and straightforward and allows your doctor to screen for diabetes sooner and work with you to manage diabetes efficiently and prevent complications.

Your doctor will use the A1C test, the fasting plasma glucose (FPG) test, or the random plasma glucose RPG test to diagnose diabetes.

- **The A1C Test and Diabetes**

The A1C test (also called hemoglobin A1C or HbA1c test) is a blood test that measures the average levels of your blood sugar over the past two to three months. The A1C test is one of the commonly used tests to diagnose the risk of prediabetes or type 2 diabetes. The A1C test is the main tool for diabetes management, as patients use it to achieve their individual A1C goals.

How does the test work?

The A1C (HbA1c) test measures the amount of sugar in your blood that is attached to hemoglobin, a protein inside your red blood cells that carries oxygen. When sugar enters your bloodstream, it binds with hemoglobin. The A1C (HbA1c) test measures the percentage of your red blood cells that are coated with glucose. Thus, a higher A1C (HbA1c) level indicates poor blood glucose control and warns of an elevated risk of developing severe diabetes complications.

If you have a diabetes condition, you should get an A1C (HbA1c) test at least twice a year to make sure diabetes is under close control and your blood glucose is in your target range.

Interpreting the A1C results

A normal A1C (HbA1c) level is under 5.7%. In healthy people, the normal range for the A1c (HbA1c) level is in the range of 4% to 5.6%

A level of A1C (HbA1c) in the range of 5.7% to 6.4% indicates prediabetes and a higher chance of developing diabetes.

A level of A1C (HbA1c) equal to or high than 6.5% indicates diabetes.

- **The fasting plasma glucose (FPG) test**

The fasting blood sugar test measures your blood glucose after an overnight fast. It's a simple, safe, and quick way to screen for prediabetes, type1, type 2 diabetes, or gestational diabetes. If you have a fasting blood sugar test scheduled, don't eat or drink anything for 8 to 12 hours before the test.

How does the test work?

When fasting, the pancreas hormone called glucagon is stimulated and causes the liver to release glucose into the bloodstream, which increases the body's blood glucose levels. If you don't have diabetes, your body will release insulin to burn excess glucose and rebalance the increased glucose levels. If you have diabetes or prediabetes, your body cannot produce enough insulin or cannot use appropriately released insulin, causing blood glucose levels will remain high. Thus, a higher fasting plasma glucose level indicates poor blood glucose control and warns of an elevated risk of diabetes or prediabetes depending on the test results.

Interpreting the FPG results

A fasting blood glucose level less than or equal to 99 mg/dL is considered normal.

A fasting blood glucose level in the range of 100 to 125 mg/dL indicates you have prediabetes and a higher chance of developing diabetes.

A fasting blood glucose level high than or equal to 126 mg/dL indicates you have diabetes.

- **Glucose Tolerance Test**

The Glucose Tolerance Test (OGTT) is used to test how your body moves glucose from the blood into the body's tissues. You then drink a liquid that contains glucose and get your blood measured. You'll fast overnight before taking the test and have your blood tested to assess your fasting blood glucose level.

Then you will drink the glucose-containing liquid and have your blood glucose level checked after 1 hour and 2 hours afterward.

Interpreting the OGTT results

At 2 hours test, a blood sugar level less than or equal to 140 mg/dL or lower is considered normal.

A blood sugar level in the range of 140 to 199 mg/dL indicates you have prediabetes and a higher risk of diabetes.

A blood sugar level high or equal to 200 mg/dL indicates you have diabetes.

- **Random Blood Sugar Test**

The random blood sugar RPG test is sometimes used to diagnose diabetes when symptoms are present and when your doctor may need to screen for diabetes without waiting until you have fasted. You may take the RPG blood test at any time. An RPG blood glucose level high than or equal to 200 mg/dL indicates you have diabetes.

13
DIABETES COMPLICATIONS

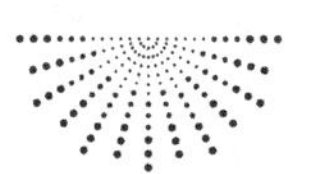

Over time, having an excess of sugar in your blood can cause complications ranging from mild to severe. Diabetes complications are often interrelated, share the same contributing causes, and combine in a dangerous way that may alter the overall health condition. For example, nearly 50% of all patients diagnosed with type 2 diabetes have high blood pressure (hypertension), which may constrict and narrow the blood vessels throughout the body, including the nerves, the eyes, and the kidney. On the other side, having high levels of glucose in your blood for a prolonged time can harm blood vessels that supply oxygen throughout your body, including the eyes, heart, kidneys, and brain. Damages that occur can lead to severe and long-term complications.

Diabetes also induces significant quantitative changes in the amount of circulating lipids characterized by an increase in triglycerides (a type of lipid in the blood), a reduction in HDL cholesterol (good), and an increase in LDL cholesterol (bad). These changes are associated with an increased risk of heart disease and stroke.

The main complications of diabetes

Diabetes complications are long-term problems that develop gradually. Diabetes complications can lead to severe damage if untreated.

- diabetic retinopathy. People with diabetes are at risk of developing an eye disorder called retinopathy due to elevated high blood pressure. Retinopathy can affect patients' eyesight and cause partial vision loss and blindness.
- diabetic foot ulcers. Foot problems are severe diabetes complications that result from concomitant actions, including damages to the nerve and impaired blood circulation. Nerve damages known as diabetic neuropathy combined with reduced blood flow affect the feeling in your feet and make it difficult for sores and cuts to heal. In some serious cases, gangrenes develop and can lead to amputation.
- diabetic nephropathy. This severe diabetes complication is common among type 1 and types 2 diabetes patients who poorly control their blood glucose. Over time, uncontrolled diabetes can lead to irreversible damage to blood vessel clusters that filter waste and extra water out of your blood. This severe condition can lead to kidney damage and kidney failure. Your kidneys are also involved in the control of blood pressure, and such damages may cause hypertension which in turn worsens kidney diseases.
- heart disease and stroke. Over time, high blood glucose can harm blood vessels and nerves that control your heart and supply oxygen to the brain and heart. Individuals with diabetes are at higher risk of developing heart disease and strokes.
- erectile dysfunction. Poor and prolonged blood glucose control may damage nerves and small blood vessels that control the erection.
- chronic inflammatory diseases. Poorly controlled diabetes may cause damage to the whole body, trigger and worsen inflammation. In turn, inflammation causes and aggravates

insulin resistance leading to much-elevated blood glucose levels.

PART IV

MAKING SMARTER AND INFORMED FOOD CHOICES

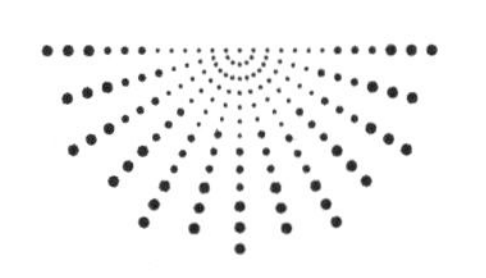

14

EATING WHOLE AND MINIMALLY PROCESSED FOODS

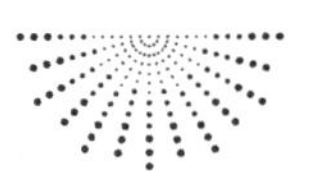

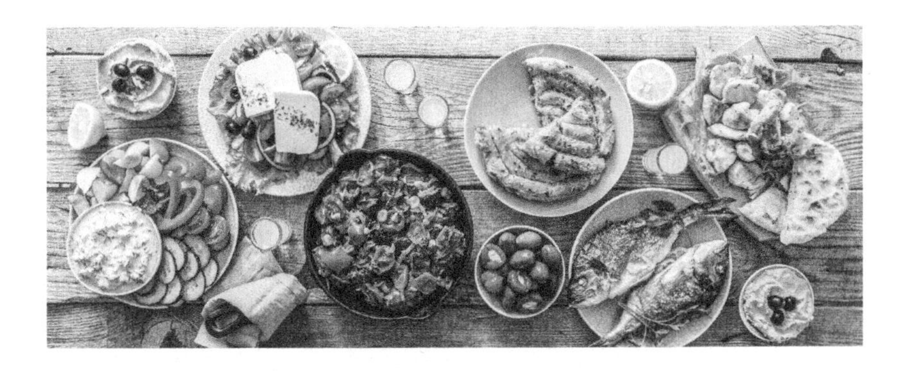

Most Americans don't eat whole foods anymore. They eat processed and highly-processed foods that are generally inferior to unprocessed or minimally processed foods. Highly-processed foods are generally industrially-made and contain many ingredients, including high-fructose corn syrup, trans fats, monosodium glutamate, artificial sweeteners, flavors, colors, and other chemical additives. Highly-processed foods are believed to be a significant contributor to the obesity epidemic in the world, promoting diabetes, chronic inflammation, and the prevalence of autoimmune diseases. Therefore, we must distinguish between healthy processed foods to include in the glycemic load for weight loss and diabetes control and those to exclude because they are considered unhealthy and pro-inflammatory.

Whole food refers to unprocessed or minimally processed food— a nature-made food without added sugars, fat, sodium, flavorings, or other artificial ingredients. It has not been broken down by man's intervention into its components and refined into a new form. Whole Foods are generally close to their natural state, unprocessed, and unrefined. Whole foods have little to no additives or preservatives.

- **The Glycemic Load Diet**

The Glycemic Load Diet is a balanced, easy, long-term, and sustainable diet that selects low glycemic, whole, or minimally processed foods and limits animal products. It mainly focuses on plants, including vegetables, fruits, whole grains, legumes, seeds, and nuts, which should make up most of what you eat. You then have to design your eating plan around **unprocessed and minimally processed foods** and, as much as you can, **avoid foods that are processed** and **absolutely exclude highly processed**.

The Glycemic Load Diet supplies your body with low glycemic, unprocessed, or minimally processed foods, with little to no unhealthy added constituents. You don't have to focus on calorie, protein, fat, or carb counting. Instead, you have to concentrate on eating foods that do not cause high blood sugar spikes and battle inflammation.

The importance of glycemic load component is critical because one can adopt a whole foods diet and still end up eating unhealthy carbohydrates-containing foods or fatty foods. Merely avoiding processed and refined foods is not the answer to better glycemic control, diabetes complications prevention, and inflammation reduction.

Frequently eating carbohydrates-containing foods that cause high spikes in your blood sugar may make it harder to control your blood sugar and put you at increased risk of diabetes complications.

Coconut, coconut oil, palm kernel oil, and palm oil fall in the category of whole foods but are full of saturated fats. Many experts, including the American Diabetes Association, and the American Heart Association, claim that replacing foods high in saturated fat with healthier alternatives may lower LDL cholesterol and triglycerides in the blood. In addition, oils rich in saturated fats are associated with increased inflammation and chronic diseases.

Thus the glycemic load component is critical to addressing such problems and providing a robust solution to achieve a healthy weight or win against diabetes.

15
EATING LOW GLYCEMIC LOAD AND ANTI-INFLAMMATORY FOODS

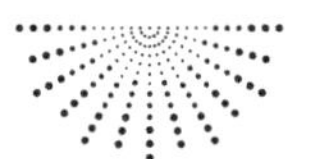

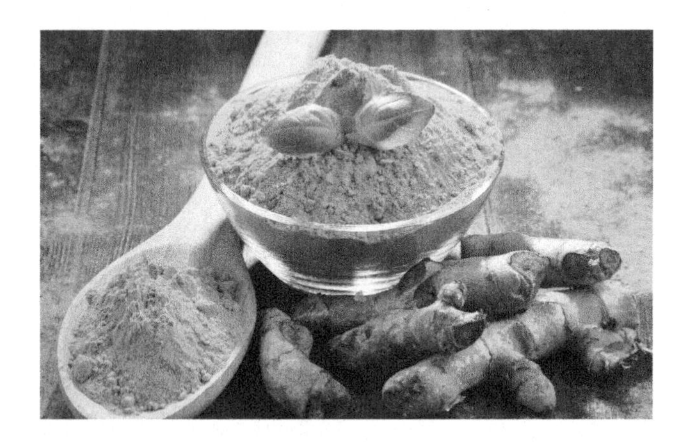

Growing lines of evidence indicate that various dietary polyphenols and flavonoids positively influence blood sugar at different levels, help control and prevent diabetes complications. Antioxidants also play a beneficial and protective role of the pancreatic beta-cells against glucose toxicity in diabetic patients. Thus, consuming polyphenols-rich foods, flavonoids-rich foods, and antioxidants will help you closely lose weight, control your blood sugar levels, and reduce the risk of developing chronic inflammatory diseases.

- **1. Eating low glycemic index vegetables and fruits**

In the glycemic load diet, you have to eat low glycemic load fruits and vegetables to avoid high spikes in your blood sugar. In addition, non-starchy vegetables and fruits are good sources of anti-inflammatory nutrients such as polyphenols, antioxidants, and flavonoids.

The serving sizes for low glycemic index vegetables and fruits are equivalent to:

- 1 cup raw or salad vegetables
- 1/2 cup cooked vegetables
- 3/4 cup (6oz) vegetable juice homemade and unsweetened
- ½ cup of cooked beans, lentils, and peas
- 1 medium piece of fruit
- 1 cup (6 oz) of sliced fruits
- ½ cup (4 oz) of fruit juice

The total vegetable intake (per day) is equivalent to 8-10 servings. You have to vary your meals using the maximal recommended amount as follows:

- "Dark-Green Vegetables" group up to 2 servings
- "Red & Orange Vegetables" group up to 3 servings
- "Beans, Peas, Lentils" group up to 2 servings
- "Starchy Vegetables" group up to 1 serving
- "Other Vegetables" group up to 3 servings

The total fruit intake is equivalent to 2-4 servings per day.

- **2. Increasing your Omega-3 Fatty Acids Intake**

Omega-3 fatty acids belong to the polyunsaturated fats family, which are associated with beneficial health effects such as

- decreasing inflammation
- improving heart health
- supporting mental health
- decreasing liver fat
- helping in the prevention of many chronic conditions
- promoting bone health

Strategies to increase your weekly intake of omega-3 fatty acids include regularly eating omega-3-rich nuts and seeds—such as chia seed, flaxseed, Hemp seed—, eating fatty fish—such as salmon, sardines, anchovies, mackerel, and herring. The weekly fish intake is equivalent to 10 servings (a serving is equal to 3 to 4 ounces). So target eating 6-8 servings of fatty fish per week.

- **3. Choosing healthy fats**

The glycemic load diet is rich in omega-3 and lower in omega-6 than most diets. High levels of omega-3 combined with a low (omega-6/omega-3) are associated with many health benefits, including a significant reduction of unnecessary inflammation and diabetes complications. For example, a ratio (omega-6/omega-3) of 4/1 was correlated to a 70% reduction in mortality. So, based on recent studies, you have to keep the ratio (omega-6/omega-3) in the range of 1/1 and 4/1, which is associated with positive health outcomes.

Strategies to achieve an adequate ratio (omega-6/omega-3) include

- consuming fatty fish (e.g., sardines, mackerels, salmon, herring, anchovies) twice a week,

- consuming nuts and seeds (e.g., flax seeds, chia seeds, walnuts) twice a week.

- **4. Increasing olive oil consumption**

Recent studies have established that an extra virgin olive oil-rich diet reduces glucose levels, LDL cholesterol (bad), and triglycerides. And thus, prevents a series of illnesses that are very common among diabetic patients.

The anti-diabetes benefits of Extra Virgin Olive Oil (EVOO) increase with the daily ingested amount. A minimum of extra virgin olive oil of four tablespoons per day is necessary to provide beneficial anti-diabetes and antioxidant effects. When cooking, EVOO is an excellent choice as it has been well established that it helps reduce blood sugar levels, reduce blood pressure, lower bad cholesterol (LDL), and decrease inflammation. The nutritional composition of virgin olive is comprised of mainly

- monounsaturated fatty acids (69.2% for extra virgin olive oil), mainly Oleic acid (omega-9)
- saturated fats (15.4% for extra virgin olive oil) mainly Stearic acid and Palmitic Acid
- polyunsaturated (9.07% for extra virgin olive oil), mainly Linoleic acid (omega-3)
- Polyphenols
- Vitamin E, Carotenoids, and Squalene

Strategies to increase your daily intake of olive oil include

- replacing butter with EVOO,
- using olive oil as finishing oil for your meals,
- replacing the oil you use for cooking,

- roasting, and frying with EVOO.

- **5. Including anti-inflammatory spices in your eating plan**

Over the several last decades, extensive research has revealed that some spices and their active components exhibit tremendous weight loss and anti-inflammatory benefits. Some spices have been found to prevent or decrease the severity of diabetes complications as well as a number of chronic conditions such as arthritis, asthma, multiple sclerosis, cardiovascular diseases, lupus, cancer, and neurodegenerative diseases. The most common spices used for their anti-inflammatory activities are

- turmeric,
- green tea,
- garlic,
- ginger,
- cayenne pepper,
- black pepper,
- black cumin,
- clove,
- cumin,
- ginseng,
- cardamom,
- parsley
- cinnamon,
- rosemary,
- chives,
- basil,
- cilantro

In addition, spices have a unique property to add flavor to any meal without adding fats or salt. Therefore, you should consider integrating herbs as part of your daily diet when cooking.

Some strategies for getting more herbs and spices in your diet include

- using some fresh herbs as the main ingredient (e.g., herb salad, tabbouleh salad),
- replacing some green vegetables in salads with herbs,
- substituting (or reducing) salt in a recipe with spices,
- replacing mayonnaise with basil-olive oil preparation,
- drinking 3–4 cups of green tea daily.

- **6. Drinking more water**

Water is critical for life. Without water, there is no life. All of the organs of our body, such as the heart, brain, lungs, and muscles, contain a significant quantity of water and need water to stay healthy.

Every day we lose water, and we need to replace it through a regular water supply. Otherwise, we can suffer from dehydration, which may alter the normal body's functions.

The recommended water intake for men aged 19+ is 3 liters (13 cups), and for women aged 19+ is 2.2 liters (9 cups) each day.

16

AVOIDING HIGH GLYCEMIC LOAD AND INFLAMMATORY FOODS

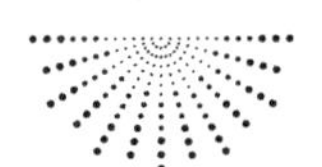

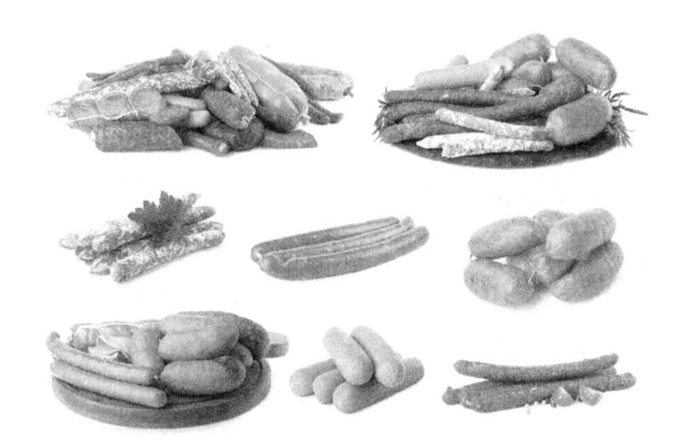

- **1. Limiting moderate glycemic load foods and avoiding high glycemic load foods**

One unit of GL corresponds to the glycemic effect of ingesting 1 g of glucose. Typical low glycemic load diets contain from 80–150 GL units per day.

For a standard serving size of food, glycemic load (GL) is considered high with GL greater or equal to 20, medium with GL in the range of 11-19, and low with GL less or equal to 10. The Daily GL is the sum of the GL values for all foods consumed during the day.

Because there is a gap in the GL ranges, a food with a glycemic load (GL) of 10.1 is considered a medium GL. A food with a glycemic load (GL) of 19.1 is considered a High GL.

Eating frequently many high glycemic load foods is associated with an increased risk for type 2 diabetes, cardiovascular disease, overweight, and obesity. Conversely, eating low glycemic load foods has been shown to help control type 2 diabetes, improve blood markers and improve weight loss.

Tables of foods with their glycemic load divided into the 14 categories are available in part VII, "Glycemic Index Counter":

- Beef, Lamb, Veal, Pork & Poultry
- Beverages
- Bread & Bakery Products
- Breakfast Cereals
- Dairy Products & Alternatives
- Soups, Pasta, and Noodles
- Fish & Fish Products
- Fruit and Fruit Products
- Legumes and Nuts
- Meat Sandwiches and Ham
- Mixed Meals and Convenience Foods
- Recipe
- Snack Foods and Confectionery
- Vegetables

- **2. Excluding Trans-Fats containing Foods**

Trans-fatty acids are mostly industrially manufactured fats produced during the hydrogenation process that adds hydrogen to liquid vegetable oils to transform the liquid to a solid form at room temperature. Trans fats give foods a desirable taste and texture. However, unlike other dietary fats, consuming trans-fatty acids raises the level of your bad cholesterol (LDL), lowers your good cholesterol (HDL) levels, increases your risk of developing severe cardiovascular conditions certain cancers, and aggravates inflammation. Trans fats may be present in several food products, including:

- fried fast foods, including french fries, fried chicken, battered fish, mozzarella sticks, and doughnuts
- margarine
- peanut butter
- baked goods (e.g. cakes, pies, and cookies made with margarine or vegetable shortening)
- vegetable shortening

Strategies to reduce drastically trans fats intake include

- avoiding or reducing intake of fried fast foods—including french fries, fried chicken, battered fish, mozzarella sticks, and doughnuts—margarine, peanut butter, frozen pizza, baked goods made with margarine or vegetable shortening
- eating smaller portion sizes
- consuming trans-fat-containing foods less frequently.

- **3. Eating a little less red meat but enough proteins**

There is little evidence that red meat may contribute to inflammation and alter glycemic control, while some recent studies revealed that unprocessed red meat might be associated with less inflammation and is safe for people with diabetes. However, there is a consensus about the danger of consuming processed red meat such as sausage, bacon, salami, and hot dogs. A 2012 study funded and supported by some health and nutrition government agencies has established the link between processed red meal consumption and increased total mortality. It also revealed that daily unprocessed red meat consumption raised the risk of total mortality by 13%. The study revealed that replacing one serving of red meat per day with other protein sources such as fish, poultry, and nuts could decrease the risk of mortality by 7-19%.

These findings suggest that you should restrict your red meat intake to reduce inflammation, and prevent and delay diabetes complications.

Eating adequate amounts of protein is extremely important for your health because proteins play a crucial role in your body's vital processes and metabolisms, such as building and repairing tissues, building muscles, blood, hair, and skin, regulating some inflammatory responses, and producing hormones, enzymes, and other body chemicals. The weekly recommended proteins intake is equivalent to

- 30 servings of animal proteins (mainly lean white meat, and eggs)
- 10 servings of seafood
- 5 servings of nuts and seeds

By restricting red meat intake in the range of 1/5 to 1/4 of animal proteins (e.g., 6 to 7.5 servings of red meat per week), you may experience improvement in your overall health and reduction of some symptoms caused by inflammation.

PART V
KNOWING WHAT IS IN THE FOOD YOU EAT

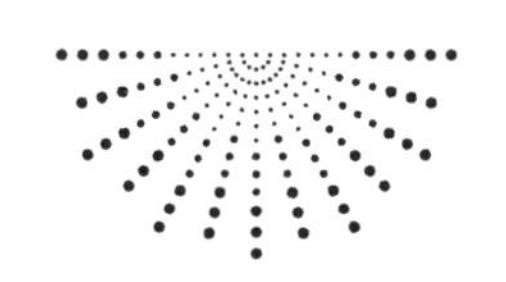

17
MASTERING CARBOHYDRATES

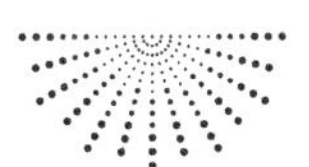

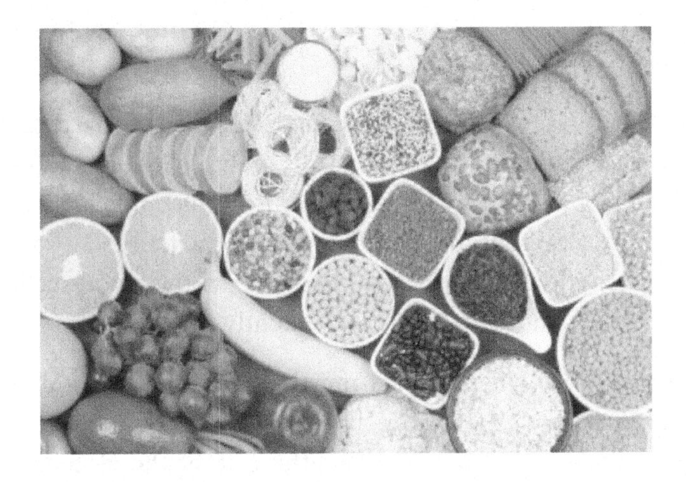

The choice of high-quality macronutrients is crucial for the success of long-term weight loss or diabetes management.

KNOWING HOW SOME HORMONES REGULATE WEIGHT

Before going deeper into the choice of healthy carbohydrates, we have to notice that you must achieve the following "Hormones balancing concepts" to achieve a healthy weight:

- **getting and maintaining the insulin down** will allow you to increase your body's insulin sensitivity and reduce any form of insulin resistance.
- **avoiding spikes in insulin level,** which is harmful to the pancreas and may induce insulin resistance, and induce increased cortisol levels —the hormone of stress— when the blood sugar decreases abruptly.
- **avoiding ultra-processed and high-processed foods** that compromise the guts' integrity and inhibit or reduce the release of leptin —the hormone of satiety.—
- **Reducing the release of ghrelin** — the hormone of hunger — by eating some nutrients that slow down the ghrelin release in the bloodstream.

UNDERSTANDING HOW CARBOHYDRATES CAN WORK FOR YOU OR AGAINST YOU

All carbohydrates, whether they are low glycemic, moderate glycemic, or high glycemic, follow the same metabolic mechanism and break down into blood sugar, which plays a crucial role in the ability of our bodies to function properly. The problem with blood sugar and consequently with carbohydrates occurs when the blood sugar levels spike high throughout the day and frequently.

These spikes arise when you eat mostly high-glycemic foods or high glycemic load foods (a notion that refers to large portion sizes of carb-containing foods). Here comes the role of the glycemic index, which doesn't refer formally to a diet in the sense that you have to conform to strict rules, follow particular meal plans or eliminate some foods from your daily meals. Instead, it's a scientific method of identifying how carbohydrates in foods affect blood sugar levels and measuring how slowly or quickly the carbohydrates in foods raise blood sugar. Thus, the Glycemic Index referential is particularly important to understand if you want to maintain weight, lose weight, take more control of diabetes, and fix some health issues.

Types of Carbohydrates in Your Diet

The primary and main function of carbohydrates is to provide energy to the human body. Dietary carbohydrates can be divided into three major categories:

- Sugars: Short-chain carbs found in foods such as fructose, glucose, sucrose, and galactose.
- Starches: Long-chain of glucose molecules, which get transformed into glucose during digestion.
- Fibers: are divided into soluble and insoluble.

Carbohydrates can also be divided according to their chemical composition into simple and complex carbs:

- Complex carbohydrates are formed by sugar molecules that are linked together in complex and long chains. Complex carbs are found in vegetables, fruits, peas, beans, and whole grains and contain natural fiber. These types of food are healthy.
- Simple carbohydrates are transformed quickly by the body and induce an increased sugar blood level. They are found in high amounts in processed foods and refined sugars. The consumption of this type of carbs is associated with health problems like type 2 diabetes, obesity, and metabolism problem. Simple carbs foods are also deprived of essential nutrients and vitamins.

Choosing the best carbohydrates

Achieving your goals in weight loss, weight maintenance, or diabetes management depends on adapting your eating plan to make the insulin, leptin, and ghrelin hormones work for you. The quality of the carbohydrates you ingest is essential in adjusting the level of the hormones. For instance, low-quality carbs (high glycemic foods) are quickly digested and lead to blood sugar spikes, which will play against you and may cause weight gain, obesity, insulin resistance, and increased cortisol levels. Conversely, the soluble and insoluble fibers in whole foods (low glycemic foods) are known to offset glucose conversion, prevent higher insulin supplies, and avoid irregular blood sugar variations that induce an excess of cortisol.

Low glycemic index foods are known for their ability to release glucose in the blood slowly and regularly. Conversely, Foods that have a high glycemic index are known for their property to release glucose rapidly. Researches suggest that foods with a low glycemic index (LGi foods) are ideal for weight loss diets and foster weight loss, in addition to their positive effect on the pancreas (insulin release), eyes, and kidney.

The glycemic index (GI) is formed on a scale from 1 to 100. Each food gets a score on this scale according to experimental data. A lower score indicates that food takes a long time to raise blood sugar levels.

18

UNDERSTANDING PROTEINS

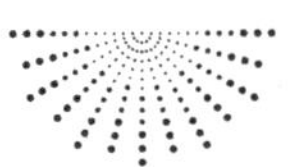

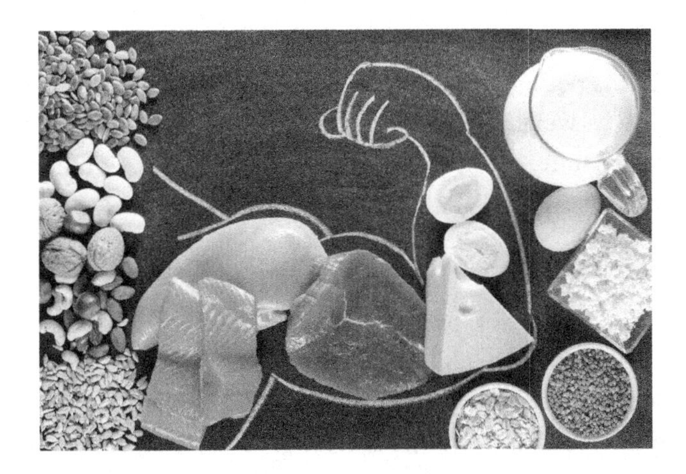

Protein is one of the three types of macronutrients present in food. Eating adequate amounts of protein is extremely important for your health because it plays a crucial role in your body's vital processes and metabolisms, such as building and repairing tissues, building muscles, blood, hair, and skin, and producing hormones, enzymes, and other body chemicals.

Unlike fats and carbs, the human body does not store protein, and you need to eat the necessary amount to keep the right hormonal balance and a healthy body. For example, when you eat protein, it transforms into amino acids, which intervene in various processes such as muscle regeneration, muscle building, and immune function regulation.

Plus, eating protein reduces levels of ghrelin (the hunger hormone) and stimulates the production of the satiety hormones (PYY and GLP-1)

Guidelines for individualized protein intake

The RDA (international Recommended Dietary Allowance) for protein is 0.8 g per kg of body weight, regardless of age. This recommendation is derived as the minimum amount to maintain nitrogen balance; however, it is not optimized for women's needs or physical activity levels.

Considering different parameters, we recommend a protein intake of 1.4-1.8 grams per kg of your body weight. Going to 1.9 grams per kg of your body weight in the premenstrual phase may be the right choice if you suffer from troubles associated with period approaches (for women).

The Protein Quality

The optimal source of protein is based on the calculation of the PDCAA (Protein Digestibility Corrected Amino Acid) Score or the DIAA (Digestibility Indispensable Amino Acid) Score. Thus, animal-based foods are identified as a superior source of protein because they offer a complete composition of essential amino acids, with higher bioavailability and digestibility (>90%).

Collagen, an essential ingredient

Collagen is the most abundant type of protein in the human body. Ligaments, tendons, skin, hair, nails, discs, and bones are collagen.

During the normal aging process, your body begins to experience a decline in the synthesis of collagen proteins. According to studies, this decline in collagen production starts around 30, at a rate of 1% per year. At the age of fifty, the rate jump to up to 3%, causing health issues:

- Muscle stiffness
- Aging joint
- Wrinkles and fine lines
- Lack of tone
- Aging skin
- Healing of wounds slower
- Frequent fatigue.

Consuming more collagen will boost your body's collagen protection. So we recommend that your daily intake of collagen represent 25 to 35% of protein.

The beneficial effects include, intestinal health, less articular pain, less hair loss, better skin, increased muscle mass

Foods rich in collagen

Here are some of the best collagen-containing foods you can add to your diet:

Bone broth

Prepared by simmering bones, ligaments, tendons, and skin of beef, bone broth is an excellent source of collagen, as well as several essential amino acids. It is also available in powder, bar, or even capsules for a collagen food supplement that is easy to add to your diet.

Spirulina

This kind of seaweed offers an excellent source of plant-based amino acids, which are key components of collagen.

Codfish

Codfish, like most other types of white fish, is a good source of collagen in addition to selenium, vitamin B6 and phosphorus.

Eggs

Eggs are a good source of collagen, including glycine and proline.

Gelatin

Gelatin is one of the best collagen-rich foods available. This is why it is advised to include it in your weight-loss diet.

19

GOOD FATS AND BAD FATS

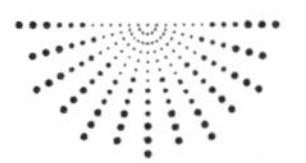

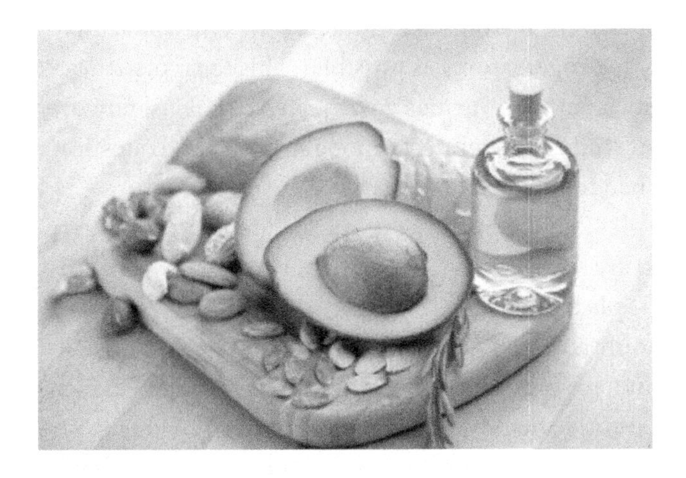

Fat is an essential macronutrient present in food, so you must understand the following information to guide you throughout your diet journey.

What is fat, and why it is essential for your health?

Dietary fats are found in both animals and vegetables and are essential for your living since they provide your body energy and support cell growth.

Fats also provide some valuable benefits and play essential roles, including:

- Help your body absorb specific nutrients like vitamins A, D, E, and K.
- Help your body produce the necessary hormones.
- Regulate inflammation and immunity issues.
- Maintain the health of your body's cells (e.g., skin, hair cells)

How many different fats are there?

There are four major fats in food, based on their chemical structures and physical properties:

- Saturated fat (bad fat): is a kind of fat in which the fatty acid chain of carbon atoms is saturated with hydrogens (holds as many hydrogen atoms as possible). This form of saturated fat is associated with various adverse health effects, however recent studies moderate the popular belief and question about how bad they impact health.
- Trans fat (bad fat): (trans-unsaturated fatty acids or trans fatty acids) are a form of unsaturated fat associated with various adverse health effects
- Monounsaturated fats (healthy fat): are a type of unsaturated fat but have only one double bond. These fats are associated with positive health effects and may replace bad fats. Monounsaturated fats are found in olive oil, avocados, and some nuts)
- Polyunsaturated fat (healthy fat): The two major classes of polyunsaturated fats are omega-3 and omega-6 fatty acids

What is cholesterol?

Cholesterol is a fat-like and waxy substance found in all the cells in your body. Plus, your body needs some cholesterol to produce steroid hormones, vitamin D, and bile acid that helps you digest fats.

Contrary to popular belief, your body makes all the cholesterol it needs in the liver. Cholesterol is supplied in small quantities (less than 15%) by plant and animals foods.

More than 85% of the cholesterol in your bloodstream comes from your liver rather than from the food you eat. Dietary cholesterol has little impact on raising blood cholesterol levels, which is valuable information from a diet perspective.

While a high cholesterol level in the blood can be dangerous, maintaining the right balance of cholesterol is essential for your health.

What types of fat should you eat?

We recommend eating fats found naturally in food and not been processed.

Several healthy sources of fat exist, such as:

- Butter and ghee (clarified butter)
- Cream
- Cheese
- Avocado (the fruit or avocado oil)
- Coconut (meat, cream, oil, milk, butter)
- Cacao butter
- Duck fat
- Medium-chained triglyceride (MCT) oil
- Pepperoni/salami/prosciutto
- Bacon fat/lard Beef
- Sardines, anchovies
- Salmon
- Olives and olive oil
- Macadamias and macadamia oil
- Almonds, Brazil nuts, hazelnuts, pecans

What Are Fatty Acids?

Fatty acids are a form of hydrocarbon chains with carboxyl at one end and methyl at the other. The biological activity of fatty acids is determined by the length of their carbon chain and their double bonds' number and position.

Saturated fatty acid does not have double bonds within the acyl chain, unsaturated fatty acid includes at least one double bond.

When two or more double bonds are present in their chain, unsaturated fatty acids are referred to as Dietary polyunsaturated fatty acids (PUFAs) and have been associated with cholesterol-lowering properties. The two families of PUFA are omega-3 and omega-6.

What Are Omega-3 Fatty Acids?

Omega-3 fatty acid is a kind of polyunsaturated fat that the human body can't produce. Thus, you need to get these essential fats from your diet.

There are various types of omega-3 fats, which differ in their chemical structure. The three most common types of omega-3 are :

- Eicosapentaenoic acid (EPA)
- Docosahexaenoic acid (DHA)
- Alpha-linolenic acid (ALA)

Omega-3 fats play a crucial role in your body:

- Improves heart health
- Supports mental health
- Reduces weight and waist size
- Decreases liver fat
- Supports infant brain development
- Fights inflammation
- Prevents dementia
- Promotes bone health

Omega-3 are essential fats that you must integrate into your weight-loss diet or the anti-inflammatory diet. They have significant benefits for your heart, brain, and metabolism.

What Are Omega-6 Fatty Acids?

Like omega-3, omega-6 fatty acids belong to the polyunsaturated fatty acids family. The omega-6 fatty acid is primarily used for energy, so you need to get it from your diet in the right quantities.

Following different recommendations and guidelines, we recommend a ratio of 4/1 omega-6 to omega-3 or less, which means that for 400 milligrams of omega-6, you have to consume 100 milligrams of omega-3. However, the Western diet has a very high ratio between 10/1 and 50/1.

Why and how is the excess of omega-6 harmful?

A high amount of omega-6 polyunsaturated fatty acids associated with a very high ratio of omega-6/omega-3 is a constant in most Western diets, including the keto diet. That increases the pathogenesis of several diseases, such as cancer, cardiovascular disease, autoimmune and inflammatory diseases. Conversely, high levels of omega-3 associated with a low ratio of omega-6/omega-3 induce health benefits. For example, a ratio of omega-6/omega-3 of 4/1 was correlated to a 70% reduction in mortality. The lower omega-6/omega-3 ratio in women who have breast cancer was connected to decreased risk.

This explains why the notion of the omega-6 / omega-3 ratio is essential in weight loss and health management.

Consuming fatty fish twice a week, eating whole foods, and choosing dairy products and meat from grass-fed animals can help you improve your omega-6:omega-3 ratio.

PART VI

THE GLYCEMIC LOAD MEAL PLANNING GUIDELINES

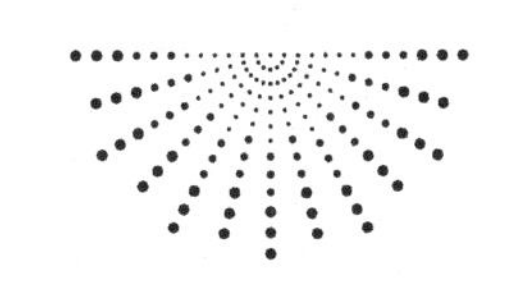

20
MEAL PLANNING GUIDELINES

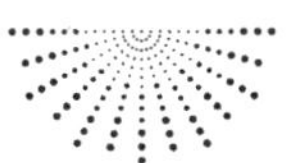

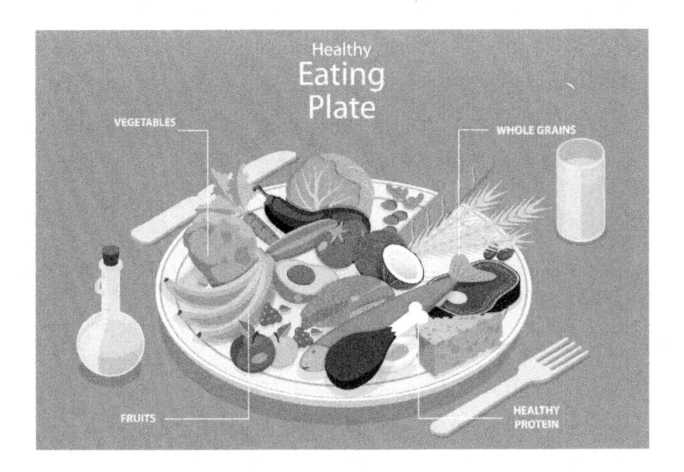

A meal plan is your guide to planning and keeping track of what you are eating. It provides clear guidelines for when, what, and how much to eat to get the sufficient nutritional elements you need while maintaining your blood glucose levels in your target range. An adequate meal plan will consider your personal goals, preferences, tastes, and lifestyle, as well as any medications you're taking.

Instead of giving strict recommendations, the dietary guidelines for diabetes give options for each food group you can choose from. Each food proposed on the different lists has anti-inflammatory properties and a low glycemic load. Following these dietary patterns will:

- help your body manage effectively blood sugar levels.
- provide adequate and sufficient nutrition with a focus on reducing risks for diabetes complications and inflammation.

All foods are also assumed to be

- unprocessed or minimally processed
- in nutrient-dense forms
- lean or low-fat
- prepared and cooked with minimal added sugars, salt (sodium), refined carbohydrates, saturated fat, or trans fats.

Recommended amounts of foods in each food group are given to allow you to design your weekly and monthly eating plan. However, you must always keep your daily GL under 50.

The five categories of foods are:

- Vegetables
- Fruits
- Grains
- Dairy and Fortified Soy Alternatives
- Protein Foods

NOTE FOR PEOPLE WITH DIABETES:

In a 2,000-calorie diet, you can eat up to 50 grams of sugar from all sources per day. This means that you should target a GL of 50—which corresponds to 50 grams of sugar.

21
VEGETABLES AND VEGETABLES PRODUCTS

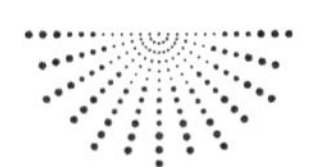

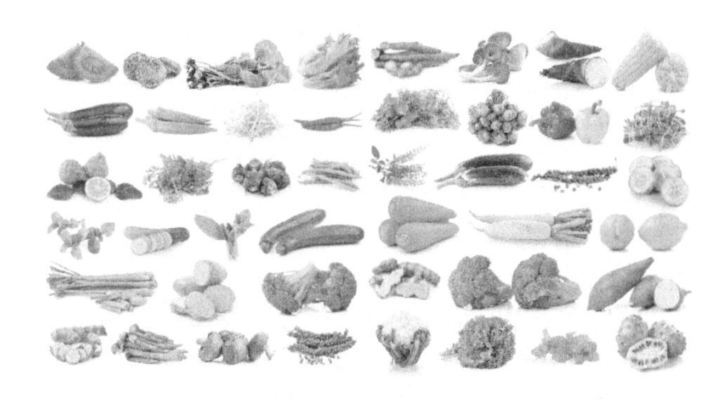

1.1 WHAT IS THE PORTION SIZE?

The typical serving sizes for vegetables and vegetable juices are equivalent to:

- 1 cup raw or salad vegetables
- 1/2 cup cooked vegetables
- 3/4 cup (6 oz) vegetable juice homemade and unsweetened
- ½ cup of cooked beans, lentils, and peas

How Much a Day?

Total vegetable intake: up to 10 servings

- "Dark-Green Vegetables" group up to 2 servings
- "Red & Orange Vegetables" group up to 3 servings
- "Beans, Peas, Lentils" group up to 2 servings
- "Starchy Vegetables" group up to 3 servings
- "Other Vegetables" group up to 3 servings

For most people, following the low-glycemic diet will require an increase in total vegetable intake from all five vegetable subgroups ("Dark-Green Vegetables", "Red & Orange Vegetables", "Beans, Peas, Lentils", "Starchy Vegetables", "Other Vegetables").

Strategies to increase total vegetable intake include

1. increasing the vegetable content of mixed dishes (more vegetables)
2. adding vegetables to breakfast
3. blending and consuming vegetables into smoothies
4. preparing sauces with vegetables
5. consuming regularly vegetable-based soups

- **Dark-Green Vegetables: The Simplified List**

- **amaranth leaves** (all fresh, frozen, cooked, or raw)
- **arugula (rocket)** (all fresh, frozen, cooked, or raw)
- **bok choy (Chinese chard)** (all fresh, frozen, cooked, or raw)
- **dandelion greens** (all fresh, frozen, cooked, or raw)
- **kale** (all fresh, frozen, cooked, or raw)
- **mustard greens** (all fresh, frozen, cooked, or raw)

- **rapini (broccoli raab)** (all fresh, frozen, cooked, or raw)
- **swiss chard** (all fresh, frozen, cooked, or raw)
- **turnip greens** (all fresh, frozen, cooked, or raw)
- **broccoli** (all fresh, frozen, cooked, or raw)
- **chamnamul** (all fresh, frozen, cooked, or raw)
- **chard** (all fresh, frozen, cooked, or raw)
- **collards** (all fresh, frozen, cooked, or raw)
- **poke greens** (all fresh, frozen, cooked, or raw)
- **romaine lettuce** (all fresh, frozen, cooked, or raw)
- **spinach** (all fresh, frozen, cooked, or raw)
- **taro leaves** (all fresh, frozen, cooked, or raw)
- **watercress** (all fresh, frozen, cooked, or raw)

- **Red and Orange Vegetables: The Simplified List**

- **acorn squash** (all fresh, frozen, vegetables or juice, cooked or raw)
- **butternut squash** (all fresh, frozen, vegetables or juice, cooked or raw)
- **calabaza** (all fresh, frozen, vegetables or juice, cooked or raw)
- **carrots** (all fresh, frozen, vegetables or juice, cooked or raw)
- **red bell peppers** (all fresh, frozen, vegetables or juice, cooked or raw)
- **hubbard squash** (all fresh, frozen, vegetables or juice, cooked or raw)
- **orange bell peppers** (all fresh, frozen, vegetables or juice, cooked or raw)
- **sweet potatoes** (all fresh, frozen, vegetables or juice, cooked or raw)
- **tomatoes** (all fresh, frozen, vegetables or juice, cooked or raw)
- **pumpkin** (all fresh, frozen, vegetables or juice, cooked or raw)
- **winter squash** (all fresh, frozen, vegetables or juice, cooked or raw)

Beans, Peas, Lentils: The Simplified List

- **beans** (all cooked from dry)
- **peas** (all cooked from dry)
- **chickpeas (Garbanzo Beans)** (all cooked from dry)
- **lentils** (all cooked from dry)
- **black beans** (all cooked from dry)
- **black-eyed peas** (all cooked from dry)
- **Bayo beans** (all cooked from dry)
- **cannellini beans** (all cooked from dry)
- **great northern beans** (all cooked from dry)
- **edamame** (all cooked from dry)
- **kidney beans** (all cooked from dry)
- **lentils** (all cooked from dry)
- **lima beans** (all cooked from dry)
- **mung beans** (all cooked from dry)
- **pigeon peas** (all cooked from dry)
- **pinto beans** (all cooked from dry)
- **split peas** (all cooked from dry)

Starchy Vegetables: The Simplified List

- **breadfruit** (all fresh, or frozen)
- **burdock root** (all fresh, or frozen)
- **cassava** (all fresh, or frozen)
- **jicama** (all fresh, or frozen)
- **lotus root** (all fresh, or frozen)
- **plantains** (all fresh, or frozen)
- **salsify** (all fresh, or frozen)
- **taro root (dasheen or yautia)** (all fresh, or frozen)
- **water chestnuts** (all fresh, or frozen)

- **yam** (all fresh, or frozen)
- **yucca** (all fresh, or frozen)

Other Vegetables: The Simplified List

- **asparagus** (all fresh, frozen, cooked, or raw)
- **avocado** (all fresh, frozen, cooked, or raw)
- **bamboo shoots** (all fresh, frozen, cooked, or raw)
- **beets** (all fresh, frozen, cooked, or raw)
- **bitter melon** (all fresh, frozen, cooked, or raw)
- **Brussels sprouts** (all fresh, frozen, cooked, or raw)
- **green cabbage** (all fresh, frozen, cooked, or raw)
- **savoy cabbage** (all fresh, frozen, cooked, or raw)
- **red cabbage** (all fresh, frozen, cooked, or raw)
- **cactus pads** (all fresh, frozen, cooked, or raw)
- **cauliflower** (all fresh, frozen, cooked, or raw)
- **celery** (all fresh, frozen, cooked, or raw)
- **chayote (mirliton)** (all fresh, frozen, cooked, or raw)
- **cucumber** (all fresh, frozen, cooked, or raw)
- **eggplant** (all fresh, frozen, cooked, or raw)
- **green beans** (all fresh, frozen, cooked, or raw)
- **kohlrabi** (all fresh, frozen, cooked, or raw)
- **luffa** (all fresh, frozen, cooked, or raw)
- **mushrooms** (all fresh, frozen, cooked, or raw)
- **okra** (all fresh, frozen, cooked, or raw)
- **onions** (all fresh, frozen, cooked, or raw)
- **radish** (all fresh, frozen, cooked, or raw)
- **rutabaga** (all fresh, frozen, cooked, or raw)
- **seaweed** (all fresh, frozen, cooked, or raw)
- **snow peas** (all fresh, frozen, cooked, or raw)
- **summer squash** (all fresh, frozen, cooked, or raw)
- **tomatillos** (all fresh, frozen, cooked, or raw)

22

FRUITS AND FRUITS PRODUCTS

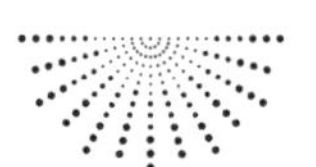

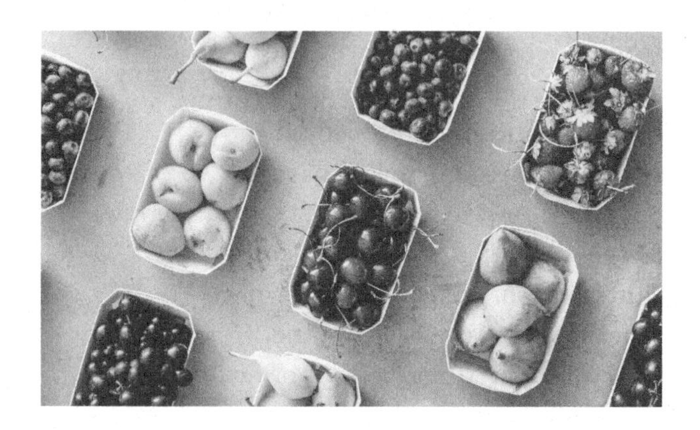

Having diabetes does not imply you can't eat fruit. The majority of fruit and vegetables are nutrient-dense, low-calorie, and packed full of essential nutrients such as vitamins, minerals, and fiber.

2.1 WHAT IS THE PORTION SIZE?

The typical serving sizes for fruits and fruits juices are equivalent to:

- 1 medium piece

- 1 cup (6 oz) of sliced fruits
- 3/4 cup (6 oz) of fruit juice

How Much a Day?

2 to 4 servings per day

The fruit food group comprises whole fruits and fruit products (100% fruit juice). Whole fruits can be eaten in various forms, such as cut, cubed, sliced, or diced. At least 60% of the recommended amount of total fruit should come from whole fruit, rather than 100% juice. Juices should be without added sugars or food additives.

For most people, following the low-glycemic diet will require an increase in total fruit. Strategies to increase total fruit intake include

1. consuming often fruits and in a variety:
2. adding fruits to breakfast.
3. choosing more whole fruits as snacks
4. blending and consuming fruits into smoothies
5. choosing and carrying fruit with you to eat later
6. creating adequate pairings with your favorite foods

- **Fruits: The Simplified List**

- **apples** (all fresh, frozen, dried fruits or 100% fruit juices)
- **Asian pears** (all fresh, frozen, dried fruits or 100% fruit juices)
- **bananas** (all fresh, frozen, dried fruits or 100% fruit juices)
- **blackberries** (all fresh, frozen, dried fruits or 100% fruit juices)
- **blueberries** (all fresh, frozen, dried fruits or 100% fruit juices)
- **currants** (all fresh, frozen, dried fruits or 100% fruit juices)

- **huckleberries** (all fresh, frozen, dried fruits or 100% fruit juices)
- **kiwifruit** (all fresh, frozen, dried fruits or 100% fruit juices)
- **mulberries** (all fresh, frozen, dried fruits or 100% fruit juices)
- **raspberries** (all fresh, frozen, dried fruits or 100% fruit juices)
- **strawberries** (all fresh, frozen, dried fruits or 100% fruit juices)
- **calamondin** (all fresh, frozen, dried fruits or 100% fruit juices)
- **grapefruit** (all fresh, frozen, dried fruits or 100% fruit juices)
- **lemons** (all fresh, frozen, dried fruits or 100% fruit juices)
- **limes** (all fresh, frozen, dried fruits or 100% fruit juices)
- **oranges** (all fresh, frozen, dried fruits or 100% fruit juices)
- **pomelos** (all fresh, frozen, dried fruits or 100% fruit juices)
- **cherries** (all fresh, frozen, dried fruits or 100% fruit juices)
- **dates** (all fresh, frozen, dried fruits or 100% fruit juices)
- **figs** (all fresh, frozen, dried fruits or 100% fruit juices)
- **grapes** (all fresh, frozen, dried fruits or 100% fruit juices)
- **guava** (all fresh, frozen, dried fruits or 100% fruit juices)
- **lychee** (all fresh, frozen, dried fruits or 100% fruit juices)
- **mangoes** (all fresh, frozen, dried fruits or 100% fruit juices)
- **nectarines** (all fresh, frozen, dried fruits or 100% fruit juices)
- **peaches** (all fresh, frozen, dried fruits or 100% fruit juices)
- **pears** (all fresh, frozen, dried fruits or 100% fruit juices)
- **plums** (all fresh, frozen, dried fruits or 100% fruit juices)
- **pomegranates** (all fresh, frozen, dried fruits or 100% fruit juices)
- **rhubarb** (all fresh, frozen, dried fruits or 100% fruit juices)
- **sapote** (all fresh, frozen, dried fruits or 100% fruit juices)
- **soursop** (all fresh, frozen, dried fruits or 100% fruit juices)

23
GRAINS

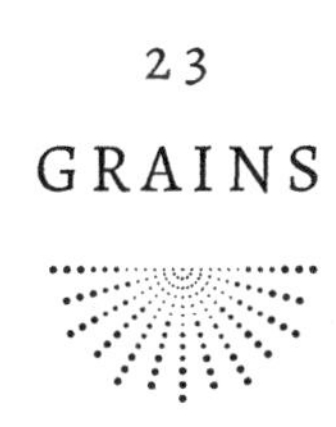

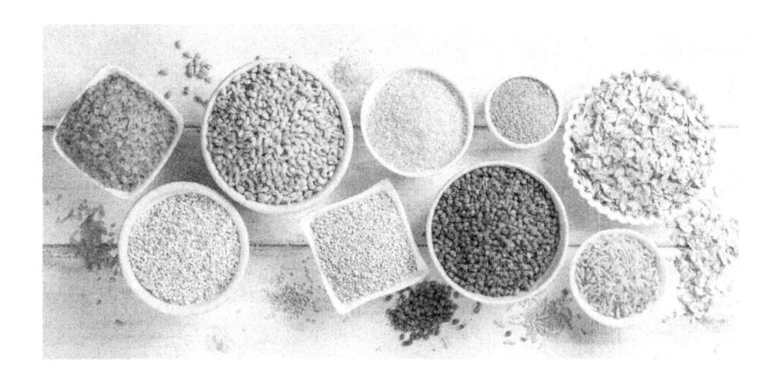

3.1 WHAT IS THE PORTION SIZE?

The typical serving sizes for cereals and grains are equivalent to:

- ⅓ cup breakfast cereal or muesli
- ½ cup of cooked cereal, or other cooked grain
- ⅓ cup of cooked rice (white rice excluded), and other small grains
- ½ cup of cold cereal

How Much a Day?

Up to 3 servings per day.

Whole grains: The Simplified List

- **barley** (all whole-grain products or used as ingredients)
- **brown rice** (all whole-grain products or used as ingredients)
- **buckwheat** (all whole-grain products or used as ingredients)
- **bulgur** (all whole-grain products or used as ingredients)
- **millet** (all whole-grain products or used as ingredients)
- **oats (Avena sativa L.)** (all whole-grain products or used as ingredients)
- **quinoa** (all whole-grain products or used as ingredients)
- **dark rye** (all whole-grain products or used as ingredients)
- **whole-wheat bread** (all whole-grain products or used as ingredients)
- **whole-wheat chapati** (all whole-grain products or used as ingredients)
- **whole-grain cereals** (all whole-grain products or used as ingredients)
- **wild rice** (all whole-grain products or used as ingredients)

24

DAIRY AND FORTIFIED SOY ALTERNATIVES

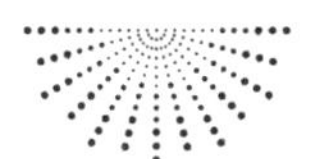

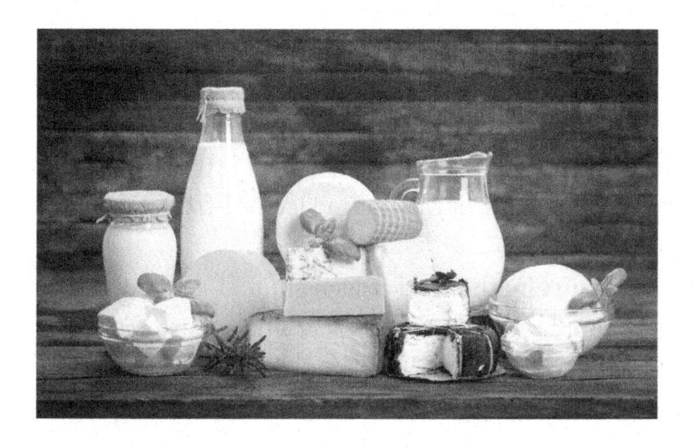

4.1 WHAT IS THE PORTION SIZE?

The typical serving sizes for dairy products are equivalent to:

- 1 cup of milk, soy beverage, or yogurt
- ⅓ cup of cottage cheese
- 1 oz of cheese

People with celiac disease or lactose intolerance should consume dairy alternatives

How Much a Day?

Up to 3 servings per day

Dairy and Fortified Soy Alternatives: The Simplified List

- **buttermilk** (all fluid, evaporated milk, or dry including lactose-free and lactose-reduced products)
- **soy beverages** (all fluid, evaporated milk, or dry including lactose-free and lactose-reduced products)
- **soy milk** (all fluid, evaporated milk, or dry including lactose-free and lactose-reduced products)
- **yogurt** (without added sugar and food additives) (all fluid, evaporated milk, or dry including lactose-free and lactose-reduced products)
- **kefir** (without added sugar and food additives) (all fluid, evaporated milk, or dry including lactose-free and lactose-reduced products)
- **frozen yogurt** (without added sugar and food additives) (all fluid, evaporated milk, or dry including lactose-free and lactose-reduced products)
- **cheeses** (all fluid, evaporated milk, or dry including lactose-free and lactose-reduced products)

25
PROTEIN FOODS

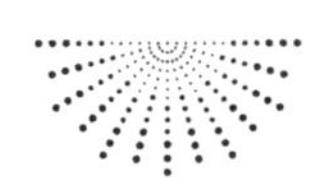

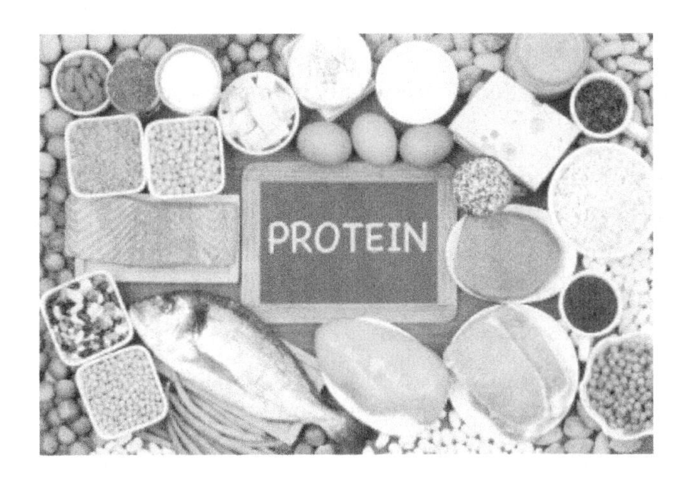

Eating adequate amounts of protein is extremely important for your health. Because Protein plays a crucial role in your body's vital processes and metabolisms, such as building and repairing tissues, building muscles, blood, hair, and skin, and producing hormones, enzymes, and other body chemicals.

Unlike carbohydrates and fat, the human body does not store protein, and you need to eat the necessary amount to keep the right hormonal balance and fight unnecessary inflammation. Animal-based foods are identified as superior sources of protein because they offer a complete composition of essential amino acids, with higher bioavailability and digestibility (>90%). Therefore, the main principle to observe here when designing your meal program is to keep a weekly proteins intake equivalent to:

- 30 servings of animal proteins (mainly lean white meat and eggs)
- 10 servings of seafood
- 5 servings of nuts and seeds

MEATS, POULTRY, EGGS, SEAFOODS: WHAT IS THE PORTION SIZE?

The typical serving sizes for the "meats, poultry, eggs", "seafood", and "nuts, seeds, soy Products" groups are equivalent to:

- 3 to 4 ounces of cooked, baked, or broiled beef
- 3 to 4 ounces of cooked, baked, or broiled veal
- 3 to 4 ounces of cooked, baked, or broiled poultry
- 3 to 4 ounces of cooked or canned fish
- 3 to 4 ounces of seafood
- 2 medium eggs
- ⅓ cup of nuts (5 large or 10 small nuts)
- 2 tablespoons of nut butter
- 2 tablespoons of nut spread

Meats, Poultry, Eggs: The simplified List

Meats (lean or low-fats) include:

- beef, goat, lamb, pork (fat red meats must be limited due to

their pro-inflammatory effects). You have to choose lean meats preferably grass-fed beef, lamb, or bison
- game meat (e.g., bison, moose, elk, deer)

Poultry (lean or low-fats) includes

- chicken
- turkey
- cornish hens
- duck
- game birds (e.g., ostrich, pheasant, and quail)
- goose.

Eggs include

- chicken eggs
- turkey eggs
- duck eggs and other birds' eggs

Seafood: The simplified List

Seafood include

- salmon
- sardine
- anchovy
- black sea bass
- catfish
- clams
- cod
- crab
- crawfish
- flounder

- haddock
- hake
- herring
- lobster
- mullet
- oyster
- perch
- pollock
- scallop
- shrimp
- sole
- squid
- tilapia
- freshwater trout
- tuna

Nuts, Seeds, Soy Products: The simplified List

Nuts (and nut butter) include

- almonds
- pecans
- Brazil nuts
- pistachios
- hazelnuts
- macadamias
- pine nuts
- walnuts
- cashew nuts

Seeds (and seed butter) include:

- pumpkin seeds

- psyllium seeds
- chia seeds.
- flax seeds
- sunflower seeds
- sesame seeds
- poppy seeds

PART VII
THE BEST FOODS (LOW GLYCEMIC LOAD FOODS)

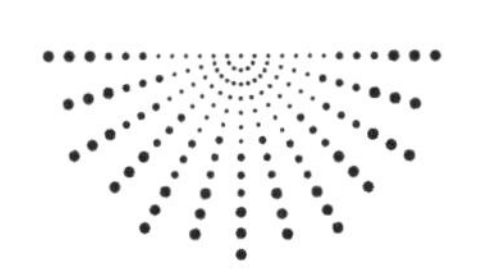

26
BAKED PRODUCTS

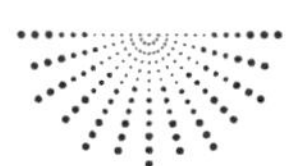

Apple Strudel ☛ Serving size= 1 oz, 28.4 g; GI= 59 (Medium); GL= 6.5 (Low); Net carb= 11 g

Bagel Multigrain ☛ Serving size= 1 miniature, 26 g; GI= 43 (Low); GL= 5 (Low); Net carb= 11.6 g

Bagel Multigrain With Raisins ☛ Serving size= 1 miniature, 26 g; GI= 49 (Low); GL= 6.1 (Low); Net carb= 12.4 g

Bagel Oat Bran ☛ Serving size= 1 miniature, 26 g; GI= 47 (Low); GL= 5.5 (Low); Net carb= 11.6 g

Bagel Pumpernickel ☛ Serving size= 1 miniature, 26 g; GI= 50 (Low); GL= 5.8 (Low); Net carb= 11.6 g

Bagel Wheat ☛ Serving size= 1 miniature, 26 g; GI= 71 (High); GL= 8.2 (Low); Net carb= 11.6 g

Bagel Wheat Bran ☛ Serving size= 1 miniature, 26 g; GI= 65 (Medium); GL= 7.5 (Low); Net carb= 11.6 g

Bagel Wheat With Fruit And Nuts ☛ Serving size= 1 miniature, 26 g; GI= 71 (High); GL= 8.6 (Low); Net carb= 12.1 g

Bagel Wheat With Raisins ☛ Serving size= 1 miniature, 26 g; GI= 71 (High); GL= 8.8 (Low); Net carb= 12.4 g

Bagel Whole Grain White ☛ Serving size= 1 miniature, 26 g; GI= 72 (High); GL= 8.4 (Low); Net carb= 11.6 g

Bagel Whole Wheat ☛ Serving size= 1 miniature, 26 g; GI= 71 (High); GL= 8.2 (Low); Net carb= 11.6 g

Bagel Whole Wheat With Raisins ☛ Serving size= 1 miniature, 26 g; GI= 71 (High); GL= 8.8 (Low); Net carb= 12.4 g

Bagel With Fruit Other Than Raisins ☛ Serving size= 1 miniature, 26 g; GI= 71 (High); GL= 8.6 (Low); Net carb= 12.1 g

Bagel, white ☛ Serving size= 1 miniature, 26 g; GI= 72 (High); GL= 9.5 (Low); Net carb= 13.2 g

Bagel, White, With Raisins ☛ Serving size= 1 miniature, 26 g; GI= 71 (High); GL= 9.8 (Low); Net carb= 13.8 g

Biscuit—Cheese ☛ Serving size= 1 biscuit (2" dia), 30 g; GI= 70 (High); GL= 9.8 (Low); Net carb= 14 g

Biscuit—Mixed Grain (Refrigerated Dough) ☛ Serving size= 1 oz, 28.4 g; GI= 70 (High); GL= 9.5 (Low); Net carb= 13.5 g

Biscuit—Plain Or Buttermilk Made From Recipe ☛ Serving size= 1 oz, 28.4 g; GI= 70 (High); GL= 8.5 (Low); Net carb= 12.2 g

Biscuit—Whole Wheat ☛ Serving size= 1 small (1-1/2" dia), 14 g; GI= 70 (High); GL= 3.9 (Low); Net carb= 5.5 g

Bread—100% Whole Grain ☛ Serving size= 1 slice, 1 oz, 28.4 g; GI= 53 (Low); GL= 5.9 (Low); Net carb= 11.2 g

Bread—Barley ☛ Serving size= 1 slice, 1 oz, 28.4 g; GI= 68 (Medium); GL= 8.5 (Low); Net carb= 12.5 g

Bread—Barley Toasted ☛ Serving size= 1 small or thin/very thin slice, 22 g; GI= 67 (Medium); GL= 7 (Low); Net carb= 10.5 g

Bread—Black Toasted ☛ Serving size= 1 oz, 28.4 g; GI= 76 (High); GL= 9.7 (Low); Net carb= 12.8 g

Bread—Buckwheat ☛ Serving size= 1 slice, 1 oz, 28.4 g; GI= 47 (Low); GL= 6.2 (Low); Net carb= 13.2 g

Bread—Cheese Toasted ☛ Serving size= 1 small or thin slice, 22 g; GI= 72 (High); GL= 7.4 (Low); Net carb= 10.3 g

Bread—Cinnamon ☛ Serving size= 1 slice, 1 oz, 28.4 g; GI= 72 (High); GL= 8.4 (Low); Net carb= 11.6 g

Bread—CornBread—Made From Recipe Made With Low Fat (2%) Milk ☛ Serving size= 1 slice, 1 oz, 28.4 g; GI= 75 (High); GL= 9.3 (Low); Net carb= 12.4 g

Bread—Cracked-Wheat ☛ Serving size= 1 slice, 1 oz, 28.4 g; GI= 73 (High); GL= 9.1 (Low); Net carb= 12.5 g

Bread—Cuban Toasted ☛ Serving size= 1 small or thin/very thin slice, 9 g; GI= 95 (High); GL= 4.7 (Low); Net carb= 4.9 g

Bread—Dough Fried ☛ Serving size= 1 slice or roll, 26 g; GI= 66 (Medium); GL= 7.5 (Low); Net carb= 11.3 g

Bread—English Muffin™ bread ☛ Serving size= 1 slice, 1 oz, 28.4 g; GI= 77 (High); GL= 8.9 (Low); Net carb= 11.5 g

Bread—Gluten-free multigrain ☛ Serving size= 1 slice, 1 oz, 28.4 g; GI= 73 (High); GL= 8.6 (Low); Net carb= 11.8 g

Bread—Italian ☛ Serving size= 1 oz, 28.4 g; GI= 70 (High); GL= 9.2 (Low); Net carb= 13.1 g

Bread—Italian Grecian Armenian ☛ Serving size= 1 small or thin/very thin slice, 24 g; GI= 70 (High); GL= 7.9 (Low); Net carb= 11.3 g

Bread—Italian Grecian Armenian Toasted ☛ Serving size= 1 small or thin/very thin slice, 22 g; GI= 70 (High); GL= 7.9 (Low); Net carb= 11.3 g

Bread—Light Rye ☛ Serving size= 1 slice, 1 oz, 28.4 g; GI= 68 (Medium); GL= 6.5 (Low); Net carb= 9.5 g

Bread—Linseed Rye ☛ Serving size= 1 slice, 1 oz, 28.4 g; GI= 55 (Medium); GL= 4.7 (Low); Net carb= 8.5 g

Bread—Marble Rye And Pumpernickel Toasted ☛ Serving size= 1 oz, 28.4 g; GI= 50 (Low); GL= 6.7 (Low); Net carb= 13.3 g

Bread—Multigrain batch ☛ Serving size= 1 slice, 1 oz, 28.4 g; GI= 63 (Medium); GL= 7.5 (Low); Net carb= 11.9 g

Bread—Oat Bran 50% ☛ Serving size= 1 slice, 1 oz, 28.4 g; GI= 44 (Low); GL= 5 (Low); Net carb= 11.4 g

Bread—Pita ☛ Serving size= 1 slice, 1 oz, 28.4 g; GI= 57 (Medium); GL= 8.7 (Low); Net carb= 15.2 g

Bread—Rice Bran ☛ Serving size= 1 oz, 28.4 g; GI= 66 (Medium); GL= 7.3 (Low); Net carb= 11 g

Bread—Rice Bran Toasted ☛ Serving size= 1 oz, 28.4 g; GI= 66 (Medium); GL= 7.9 (Low); Net carb= 11.9 g

Bread—Rice Toasted ☛ Serving size= 1 oz, 28.4 g; GI= 66 (Medium); GL= 8.6 (Low); Net carb= 13 g

Bread—Rye ☛ Serving size= 1 slice, 1 oz, 28.4 g; GI= 59 (Medium); GL= 7.8 (Low); Net carb= 13.2 g

Bread—Soy ☛ Serving size= 1 oz, 28.4 g; GI= 44 (Low); GL= 4.7 (Low); Net carb= 10.7 g

Bread—Soy Toasted ☛ Serving size= 1 oz, 28.4 g; GI= 44 (Low); GL= 5.1 (Low); Net carb= 11.7 g

Bread—Stuffing Paxo ☛ Serving size= 1 slice, 1 oz, 28.4 g; GI= 74 (High); GL= 6.1 (Low); Net carb= 8.2 g

Bread—Sunflower And Barley ☛ Serving size= 1 slice, 1 oz, 28.4 g; GI= 57 (Medium); GL= 5.2 (Low); Net carb= 9.2 g

Bread—Wholegrain pumpernickel ☛ Serving size= 1 slice, 1 oz, 28.4 g; GI= 46 (Low); GL= 3.3 (Low); Net carb= 7.2 g

Butter Croissants ☛ Serving size= 1 oz, 28.4 g; GI= 71 (High); GL= 8.7 (Low); Net carb= 12.3 g

Cake—Cherry Fudge With Chocolate Frosting ☛ Serving size= 1 oz, 28.4 g; GI= 55 (Medium); GL= 5.9 (Low); Net carb= 10.7 g

Cake—Sponge Made From Recipe ☛ Serving size= 1 oz, 28.4 g; GI= 55 (Medium); GL= 9 (Low); Net carb= 16.4 g

Churros ☛ Serving size= 1 churro, 26 g; GI= 66 (Medium); GL= 8.4 (Low); Net carb= 12.7 g

Coconut Custard Pie ☛ Serving size= 1 oz, 28.4 g; GI= 53 (Low); GL= 4.3 (Low); Net carb= 8.1 g

Coconut Macaroon (Archway Home Style Cookies) ☛ Serving size= 1 serving, 22 g; GI= 69 (Medium); GL= 8.5 (Low); Net carb= 12.3 g

Coookie—Butter Or Sugar With Fruit And/or Nuts ☛ Serving size= 1 miniature/bite size, 5 g; GI= 69 (Medium); GL= 2.2 (Low); Net carb= 3.2 g

Coookie—Butter Or Sugar With Icing Or Filling Other Than Chocolate ☛ Serving size= 1 miniature/bite size, 7 g; GI= 69 (Medium); GL= 3.5 (Low); Net carb= 5.1 g

Coookie—Chocolate Chip Made From Home Recipe Or Purchased At A Bakery ☛ Serving size= 1 miniature/bite size, 5 g; GI= 69 (Medium); GL= 1.9 (Low); Net carb= 2.8 g

Corn Flour Patty Or Tart Fried ☛ Serving size= 1 patty, 10 g; GI= 75 (High); GL= 2.9 (Low); Net carb= 3.8 g

CornBread—Made From Home Recipe ☛ Serving size= 1 surface inch, 11 g; GI= 75 (High); GL= 3.4 (Low); Net carb= 4.5 g

Cornmeal—Fritter Puerto Rican Style ☛ Serving size= 1 fritter (2-

1/2" x 2-1/2" x 1/4"), 40 g; GI= 71 (High); GL= 5.6 (Low); Net carb= 7.9 g

Crackers—Cheese Low Sodium ☛ Serving size= 1/2 oz, 14.2 g; GI= 67 (Medium); GL= 5.3 (Low); Net carb= 7.9 g

Crackers—Cheese Regular ☛ Serving size= 1/2 oz, 14.2 g; GI= 67 (Medium); GL= 5.4 (Low); Net carb= 8.1 g

Crackers—Standard Snack-Type Sandwich With Peanut Butter Filling ☛ Serving size= 1/2 oz, 14.2 g; GI= 69 (Medium); GL= 5.5 (Low); Net carb= 8 g

Crackers—Standard Snack-Type With Whole Wheat ☛ Serving size= 5 crackers 1 serving, 15 g; GI= 70 (High); GL= 6.7 (Low); Net carb= 9.5 g

Crackers—Water Biscuits ☛ Serving size= 4 cracker 1 serving, 14 g; GI= 69 (Medium); GL= 6.3 (Low); Net carb= 9.2 g

Crackers—Wheat Low Salt ☛ Serving size= 1/2 oz, 14.2 g; GI= 71 (High); GL= 6.1 (Low); Net carb= 8.6 g

Crackers—Whole-Wheat Low Salt ☛ Serving size= 1/2 oz, 14.2 g; GI= 66 (Medium); GL= 5.5 (Low); Net carb= 8.3 g

Cream Puff Shell Made From Recipe ☛ Serving size= 1 oz, 28.4 g; GI= 55 (Medium); GL= 3.4 (Low); Net carb= 6.2 g

Croissant Chocolate ☛ Serving size= 1 oz, 28.4 g; GI= 73 (High); GL= 9.6 (Low); Net carb= 13.1 g

Croissant Fruit ☛ Serving size= 1 oz, 28.4 g; GI= 71 (High); GL= 8.9 (Low); Net carb= 12.5 g

Croissants Apple ☛ Serving size= 1 oz, 28.4 g; GI= 71 (High); GL= 7 (Low); Net carb= 9.8 g

Croutons Seasoned ☛ Serving size= 1/2 oz, 14.2 g; GI= 70 (High); GL= 5.8 (Low); Net carb= 8.3 g

Crumpet ☛ Serving size= 1 small (2-1/2" dia), 20 g; GI= 73 (High); GL= 3.9 (Low); Net carb= 5.3 g

Crumpet Toasted ☛ Serving size= 1 small (2-1/2" dia), 18 g; GI= 73 (High); GL= 3.9 (Low); Net carb= 5.4 g

Danish Pastry—Cheese ☛ Serving size= 1 oz, 28.4 g; GI= 63 (Medium); GL= 6.5 (Low); Net carb= 10.3 g

Danish Pastry—Cinnamon Enriched ☛ Serving size= 1 oz, 28.4 g; GI= 63 (Medium); GL= 7.7 (Low); Net carb= 12.3 g

Danish Pastry—Cinnamon Unenriched ☛ Serving size= 1 oz, 28.4 g; GI= 63 (Medium); GL= 7.7 (Low); Net carb= 12.3 g

Danish Pastry—Fruit Enriched (Apple, Raisin, Lemon, Raisin, Raspberry, Strawberry, Cinnamon) ☛ Serving size= 1 oz, 28.4 g; GI= 63 (Medium); GL= 8.2 (Low); Net carb= 13 g

Danish Pastry—Fruit Unenriched (Apple, Raisin, Strawberry, Cinnamon) ☛ Serving size= 1 oz, 28.4 g; GI= 63 (Medium); GL= 8.2 (Low); Net carb= 13 g

Danish Pastry—Lemon Unenriched ☛ Serving size= 1 oz, 28.4 g; GI= 63 (Medium); GL= 8.2 (Low); Net carb= 13 g

Danish Pastry—Raspberry Unenriched ☛ Serving size= 1 oz, 28.4 g; GI= 63 (Medium); GL= 8.2 (Low); Net carb= 13 g

Doughnut—Yeast-Leavened Glazed Enriched (Includes Honey Buns) ☛ Serving size= 1 oz, 28.4 g; GI= 77 (High); GL= 10 (Low); Net carb= 13 g

Doughnut—Yeast-Leavened Glazed Unenriched (Includes Honey Buns) ☛ Serving size= 1 oz, 28.4 g; GI= 69 (Medium); GL= 8.4 (Low); Net carb= 12.2 g

Doughnut—Yeast-Leavened With Creme Filling ☛ Serving size= 1 oz, 28.4 g; GI= 55 (Medium); GL= 4.6 (Low); Net carb= 8.3 g

Doughnut—Yeast-Leavened With Jelly Filling ☛ Serving size= 1 oz, 28.4 g; GI= 55 (Medium); GL= 5.9 (Low); Net carb= 10.8 g

Dumpling Plain ☛ Serving size= 1 small, 18 g; GI= 63 (Medium); GL= 2.2 (Low); Net carb= 3.5 g

English Muffins ☛ Serving size= 1 oz, 28.4 g; GI= 70 (High); GL= 8 (Low); Net carb= 11.4 g

English Muffins—Mixed-Grain (Includes Granola) ☛ Serving size= 1 oz, 28.4 g; GI= 71 (High); GL= 8.8 (Low); Net carb= 12.4 g

English Muffins—Plain Enriched With Ca Prop (Includes Sourdough) ☛ Serving size= 1 oz, 28.4 g; GI= 70 (High); GL= 8.1 (Low); Net carb= 11.6 g

English Muffins—Plain Enriched (Includes Sourdough) ☛ Serving size= 1 oz, 28.4 g; GI= 72 (High); GL= 8.9 (Low); Net carb= 12.3 g

English Muffins—Plain Unenriched (Includes Sourdough), with E280 ☛ Serving size= 1 oz, 28.4 g; GI= 73 (High); GL= 9 (Low); Net carb= 12.3 g

English Muffins—Plain Unenriched (Includes Sourdough) ☛ Serving size= 1 oz, 28.4 g; GI= 73 (High); GL= 9 (Low); Net carb= 12.3 g

English Muffins—Raisin-Cinnamon (Includes Apple-Cinnamon) ☛ Serving size= 1 oz, 28.4 g; GI= 73 (High); GL= 9.4 (Low); Net carb= 12.9 g

English Muffins—Whole-Wheat ☛ Serving size= 1 oz, 28.4 g; GI= 70 (High); GL= 6.7 (Low); Net carb= 9.6 g

French Toast—Frozen—Ready-To-Heat ☛ Serving size= 1 oz, 28.4 g; GI= 79 (High); GL= 7 (Low); Net carb= 8.8 g

French Toast—Made From Recipe Made With Low Fat (2%) Milk ☛ Serving size= 1 oz, 28.4 g; GI= 79 (High); GL= 5.6 (Low); Net carb= 7.1 g

Fritter Apple ☛ Serving size= 1 fritter (2-1/2" long x 1-5/8" wide), 17 g; GI= 61 (Medium); GL= 3.5 (Low); Net carb= 5.7 g

Fritter Banana ☛ Serving size= 1 fritter (2" long), 34 g; GI= 63 (Medium); GL= 6.9 (Low); Net carb= 11 g

Fritter Berry ☛ Serving size= 1 fritter (1-1/4" dia), 24 g; GI= 61 (Medium); GL= 4.3 (Low); Net carb= 7.1 g

Leavening Agents—Baking Powder—Acting Sodium Aluminum Sulfate ☛ Serving size= 1 tsp, 4.6 g; GI= 65 (Medium); GL= 0.8 (Low); Net carb= 1.3 g

Leavening Agents—Baking Powder—Double-Acting Straight Phosphate ☛ Serving size= 1 tsp, 4.6 g; GI= 65 (Medium); GL= 0.7 (Low); Net carb= 1.1 g

Leavening Agents—Baking Powder—Low-Sodium ☛ Serving size= 1 tsp, 5 g; GI= 81 (High); GL= 1.8 (Low); Net carb= 2.2 g

Leavening Agents—Cream Of Tartar ☛ Serving size= 1 tsp, 3 g; GI= 92 (High); GL= 1.7 (Low); Net carb= 1.8 g

Leavening Agents—Yeast Bakers Active Dry ☛ Serving size= 1 tsp, 4 g; GI= 53 (Low); GL= 0.3 (Low); Net carb= 0.6 g

Leavening Agents—Yeast Bakers Compressed ☛ Serving size= 1 cake (0.6 oz), 17 g; GI= 51 (Low); GL= 0.9 (Low); Net carb= 1.7 g

Muffin—Cheese ☛ Serving size= 1 muffin, 58 g; GI= 55 (Medium); GL= 9.4 (Low); Net carb= 17 g

Muffin—Whole Grain ☛ Serving size= 1 miniature, 25 g; GI= 53 (Low); GL= 5.8 (Low); Net carb= 11 g

Muffin—Whole Wheat ☛ Serving size= 1 miniature, 25 g; GI= 51 (Low); GL= 5.2 (Low); Net carb= 10.2 g

Old Fashioned Windmill Cookies (Archway Home Style Cookies) ☛ Serving size= 1 serving, 20 g; GI= 69 (Medium); GL= 9.7 (Low); Net carb= 14.1 g

Pancake—Blueberry Made From Recipe ☛ Serving size= 1 oz, 28.4 g; GI= 67 (Medium); GL= 5.5 (Low); Net carb= 8.2 g

Pancake—Buttermilk Made From Recipe ☛ Serving size= 1 oz, 28.4 g; GI= 67 (Medium); GL= 5.5 (Low); Net carb= 8.2 g

Pancake—Plain Dry Mix Complete Made ☛ Serving size= 1 oz, 28.4 g; GI= 89 (High); GL= 9 (Low); Net carb= 10.1 g

Pancake—Plain Dry Mix Incomplete Made ☛ Serving size= 1 oz, 28.4 g; GI= 69 (Medium); GL= 5.3 (Low); Net carb= 7.7 g

Pancake—Plain Frozen—Ready-To-Heat (Includes Buttermilk) ☛ Serving size= 1 oz, 28.4 g; GI= 72 (High); GL= 7.5 (Low); Net carb= 10.4 g

Pancake—Plain Frozen—Ready-To-Heat Microwave (Includes Buttermilk) ☛ Serving size= 1 oz, 28.4 g; GI= 75 (High); GL= 8.7 (Low); Net carb= 11.6 g

Pancake—Plain Made From Recipe ☛ Serving size= 1 oz, 28.4 g; GI= 67 (Medium); GL= 5.4 (Low); Net carb= 8 g

Peanut Butter (Archway Home Style Cookies) ☛ Serving size= 1 serving, 21 g; GI= 69 (Medium); GL= 8.1 (Low); Net carb= 11.7 g

Pie Crust—Standard-Type Dry Mix ☛ Serving size= 1 oz, 28.4 g; GI= 59 (Medium); GL= 8.7 (Low); Net carb= 14.8 g

Pie Crust—Standard-Type Dry Mix Made Baked ☛ Serving size= 1 piece (1/8 of 9 inch crust), 20 g; GI= 59 (Medium); GL= 5.7 (Low); Net carb= 9.7 g

Pie Crust—Standard-Type Frozen Ready-To-Bake Enriched ☛ Serving size= 1 piece (1/8 of 9 inch crust), 18 g; GI= 59 (Medium); GL= 4.9 (Low); Net carb= 8.3 g

Pie Crust—Standard-Type Made From Recipe Baked ☛ Serving size= 1 piece (1/8 of 9 inch crust), 23 g; GI= 59 (Medium); GL= 6.2 (Low); Net carb= 10.5 g

Pie Crust—Standard-Type Made From Recipe Unbaked ☛ Serving size= 1 piece (1/8 of 9 inch crust), 24 g; GI= 59 (Medium); GL= 5.5 (Low); Net carb= 9.3 g

Pie Fried—Pies Cherry ☛ Serving size= 1 oz, 28.4 g; GI= 59 (Medium); GL= 6.7 (Low); Net carb= 11.4 g

Pie Fried—Pies Fruit ☛ Serving size= 1 oz, 28.4 g; GI= 59 (Medium); GL= 6.7 (Low); Net carb= 11.4 g

Pie Fried—Pies Lemon ☛ Serving size= 1 oz, 28.4 g; GI= 59 (Medium); GL= 6.7 (Low); Net carb= 11.4 g

Pie—Apple, Commercially Made Enriched Flour ☛ Serving size= 1 oz, 28.4 g; GI= 59 (Medium); GL= 5.4 (Low); Net carb= 9.2 g

Pie—Apple, Commercially Made Unenriched Flour ☛ Serving size= 1 oz, 28.4 g; GI= 59 (Medium); GL= 5.4 (Low); Net carb= 9.2 g

Pie—Apple Made From Recipe ☛ Serving size= 1 oz, 28.4 g; GI= 59 (Medium); GL= 6.2 (Low); Net carb= 10.5 g

Pie—Banana Cream Made From Mix No-Bake Type ☛ Serving size= 1 oz, 28.4 g; GI= 59 (Medium); GL= 5.2 (Low); Net carb= 8.8 g

Pie—Banana Cream Made From Recipe ☛ Serving size= 1 oz, 28.4 g; GI= 59 (Medium); GL= 5.4 (Low); Net carb= 9.1 g

Pie—Blueberry ☛ Serving size= 1 oz, 28.4 g; GI= 59 (Medium); GL= 5.7 (Low); Net carb= 9.6 g

Pie—Blueberry Made From Recipe ☛ Serving size= 1 oz, 28.4 g; GI= 59 (Medium); GL= 5.6 (Low); Net carb= 9.5 g

Pie—Cherry Commercially Made ☛ Serving size= 1 oz, 28.4 g; GI= 59 (Medium); GL= 6.5 (Low); Net carb= 11.1 g

Pie—Cherry Made From Recipe ☛ Serving size= 1 oz, 28.4 g; GI= 59 (Medium); GL= 6.4 (Low); Net carb= 10.9 g

Pie—Chocolate Mousse Made From Mix No-Bake Type ☛ Serving size= 1 oz, 28.4 g; GI= 59 (Medium); GL= 5 (Low); Net carb= 8.4 g

Pie—Coconut Cream Made From Mix No-Bake Type ☛ Serving size= 1 oz, 28.4 g; GI= 59 (Medium); GL= 4.7 (Low); Net carb= 8 g

Pie—Coconut Creme Commercially Made ☛ Serving size= 1 oz, 28.4 g; GI= 59 (Medium); GL= 6 (Low); Net carb= 10.2 g

Pie—Egg Custard Commercially Made ☛ Serving size= 1 oz, 28.4 g; GI= 59 (Medium); GL= 3.2 (Low); Net carb= 5.5 g

Pie—Lemon Meringue Commercially Made ☛ Serving size= 1 oz, 28.4 g; GI= 59 (Medium); GL= 7.7 (Low); Net carb= 13.1 g

Pie—Lemon Meringue Made From Recipe ☛ Serving size= 1 oz, 28.4 g; GI= 59 (Medium); GL= 6.5 (Low); Net carb= 11.1 g

Pie—Mince Made From Recipe ☛ Serving size= 1 oz, 28.4 g; GI= 59 (Medium); GL= 7.6 (Low); Net carb= 12.9 g

Pie—Peach ☛ Serving size= 1 oz, 28.4 g; GI= 59 (Medium); GL= 5.4 (Low); Net carb= 9.1 g

Pie—Pecan Commercially Made ☛ Serving size= 1 oz, 28.4 g; GI= 59 (Medium); GL= 9.6 (Low); Net carb= 16.3 g

Pie—Pecan Made From Recipe ☛ Serving size= 1 oz, 28.4 g; GI= 59 (Medium); GL= 8.7 (Low); Net carb= 14.8 g

Pie—Pumpkin Commercially Made ☛ Serving size= 1 oz, 28.4 g; GI= 59 (Medium); GL= 5.5 (Low); Net carb= 9.4 g

Pie—Pumpkin Made From Recipe ☛ Serving size= 1 oz, 28.4 g; GI= 59 (Medium); GL= 4.4 (Low); Net carb= 7.5 g

Pie—Vanilla Cream Made From Recipe ☛ Serving size= 1 oz, 28.4 g; GI= 59 (Medium); GL= 5.4 (Low); Net carb= 9.1 g

Roll—Dinner Wheat ☛ Serving size= 1 roll (1 oz), 28 g; GI= 77 (High); GL= 9.1 (Low); Net carb= 11.8 g

Roll—Dinner Whole-Wheat ☛ Serving size= 1 roll (1 oz), 28 g; GI= 77 (High); GL= 9.4 (Low); Net carb= 12.2 g

Waffle—Buttermilk Frozen—Ready-To-Heat Toasted ☛ Serving size= 1 oz, 28 g; GI= 76 (High); GL= 9.7 (Low); Net carb= 12.8 g

Waffle—Plain Frozen—Ready-To-Heat ☛ Serving size= 1 oz, 28.4 g; GI= 75 (High); GL= 8.7 (Low); Net carb= 11.6 g

Waffle—Plain Frozen—Ready-To-Heat Microwave ☛ Serving size= 1 waffle, round (4 inchdia), 32 g; GI= 71 (High); GL= 9.8 (Low); Net carb= 13.8 g

Waffle—Plain Made From Recipe ☛ Serving size= 1 oz, 28.4 g; GI= 69 (Medium); GL= 6.4 (Low); Net carb= 9.3 g

27
BEEF, LAMP, VEAL, PORK & POULTRY

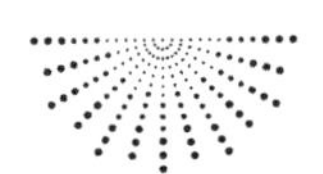

Beef-Offal—Heart ☛ Serving size= 3 oz, 85 g; GI= 0 (Low); GL= 0 (Low); Net carb= 0 g

Beef-Offal—Heart: Battered + fried ☛ Serving size= 3 oz, 85 g; GI= 0 (Low); GL= 0 (Low); Net carb= 17 g

Beef-Offal—Heart: Braised, Broiled or Baked ☛ Serving size= 3 oz, 85 g; GI= 0 (Low); GL= 0 (Low); Net carb= 0 g

Beef-Offal—Heart: Fried, Stewed or Roast ☛ Serving size= 3 oz, 85 g; GI= 0 (Low); GL= 0 (Low); Net carb= 0 g

Beef—Bottom Round ☛ Serving size= 3 oz, 85 g; GI= 0 (Low); GL= 0 (Low); Net carb= 0 g

Beef—Bottom Round: Battered + fried ☛ Serving size= 3 oz, 85 g; GI= 0 (Low); GL= 0 (Low); Net carb= 17 g

Beef—Bottom Round: Braised, Broiled or Baked ☛ Serving size= 3 oz, 85 g; GI= 0 (Low); GL= 0 (Low); Net carb= 0 g

Beef—Bottom Round: Fried, Stewed or Roast ☛ Serving size= 3 oz, 85 g; GI= 0 (Low); GL= 0 (Low); Net carb= 0 g

Beef—Brain ☛ Serving size= 3 oz, 85 g; GI= 0 (Low); GL= 0 (Low); Net carb= 0 g

Beef—Brain: Braised, Broiled or Baked ☛ Serving size= 3 oz, 85 g; GI= 0 (Low); GL= 0 (Low); Net carb= 0 g

Beef—Brain: Fried, Stewed or Roast ☛ Serving size= 3 oz, 85 g; GI= 0 (Low); GL= 0 (Low); Net carb= 0 g

Beef—Brisket ☛ Serving size= 3 oz, 85 g; GI= 0 (Low); GL= 0 (Low); Net carb= 0 g

Beef—Brisket: Battered + fried ☛ Serving size= 3 oz, 85 g; GI= 0 (Low); GL= 0 (Low); Net carb= 17 g

Beef—Brisket: Braised, Broiled or Baked ☛ Serving size= 3 oz, 85 g; GI= 0 (Low); GL= 0 (Low); Net carb= 0 g

Beef—Brisket: Fried, Stewed or Roast ☛ Serving size= 3 oz, 85 g; GI= 0 (Low); GL= 0 (Low); Net carb= 0 g

Beef—Chuck Roast ☛ Serving size= 3 oz, 85 g; GI= 0 (Low); GL= 0 (Low); Net carb= 0 g

Beef—Chuck Roast: Battered + fried ☛ Serving size= 3 oz, 85 g; GI= 0 (Low); GL= 0 (Low); Net carb= 17 g

Beef—Chuck Roast: Braised, Broiled or Baked ☛ Serving size= 3 oz, 85 g; GI= 0 (Low); GL= 0 (Low); Net carb= 0 g

Beef—Chuck Roast: Fried, Stewed or Roast ☛ Serving size= 3 oz, 85 g; GI= 0 (Low); GL= 0 (Low); Net carb= 0 g

Beef—Chuck Steak Varieties Chart ☛ Serving size= 3 oz, 85 g; GI= 0 (Low); GL= 0 (Low); Net carb= 0 g

Beef—Chuck Steak Varieties Chart: Battered + fried ☛ Serving size= 3 oz, 85 g; GI= 0 (Low); GL= 0 (Low); Net carb= 17 g

Beef—Chuck Steak Varieties Chart: Braised, Broiled or Baked ☛ Serving size= 3 oz, 85 g; GI= 0 (Low); GL= 0 (Low); Net carb= 0 g

Beef—Chuck Steak Varieties Chart: Fried, Stewed or Roast ☛ Serving size= 3 oz, 85 g; GI= 0 (Low); GL= 0 (Low); Net carb= 0 g

Beef—Cuts of Steak ☛ Serving size= 3 oz, 85 g; GI= 0 (Low); GL= 0 (Low); Net carb= 0 g

Beef—Cuts of Steak: Battered + fried ☛ Serving size= 3 oz, 85 g; GI= 0 (Low); GL= 0 (Low); Net carb= 17 g

Beef—Cuts of Steak: Braised, Broiled or Baked ☛ Serving size= 3 oz, 85 g; GI= 0 (Low); GL= 0 (Low); Net carb= 0 g

Beef—Cuts of Steak: Fried, Stewed or Roast ☛ Serving size= 3 oz, 85 g; GI= 0 (Low); GL= 0 (Low); Net carb= 0 g

Beef—Delmonico Steak ☛ Serving size= 3 oz, 85 g; GI= 0 (Low); GL= 0 (Low); Net carb= 0 g

Beef—Delmonico Steak: Battered + fried ☛ Serving size= 3 oz, 85 g; GI= 0 (Low); GL= 0 (Low); Net carb= 17 g

Beef—Delmonico Steak: Braised, Broiled or Baked ☛ Serving size= 3 oz, 85 g; GI= 0 (Low); GL= 0 (Low); Net carb= 0 g

Beef—Delmonico Steak: Fried, Stewed or Roast ☛ Serving size= 3 oz, 85 g; GI= 0 (Low); GL= 0 (Low); Net carb= 0 g

Beef—Doner Kebab ☛ Serving size= 3 oz, 85 g; GI= 85 (High); GL= 6.4 (Low); Net carb= 7.5 g

Beef—frankfurter ☛ Serving size= 1 frankfurter, 45 g; GI= 28 (Low); GL= 0.5 (Low); Net carb= 1.8 g

Beef—Hanger Steak ☛ Serving size= 3 oz, 85 g; GI= 0 (Low); GL= 0 (Low); Net carb= 0 g

Beef—Hanger Steak: Battered + fried ☛ Serving size= 3 oz, 85 g; GI= 0 (Low); GL= 0 (Low); Net carb= 17 g

Beef—Hanger Steak: Braised, Broiled or Baked ☛ Serving size= 3 oz, 85 g; GI= 0 (Low); GL= 0 (Low); Net carb= 0 g

Beef—Hanger Steak: Fried, Stewed or Roast ☛ Serving size= 3 oz, 85 g; GI= 0 (Low); GL= 0 (Low); Net carb= 0 g

Beef—Kidney ☛ Serving size= 3 oz, 85 g; GI= 0 (Low); GL= 0 (Low); Net carb= 0 g

Beef—Kidney: Braised, Broiled or Baked ☛ Serving size= 3 oz, 85 g; GI= 0 (Low); GL= 0 (Low); Net carb= 0 g

Beef—Kidney: Fried, Stewed or Roast ☛ Serving size= 3 oz, 85 g; GI= 0 (Low); GL= 0 (Low); Net carb= 0 g

Beef—Liver ☛ Serving size= 1 slice, 81 g; GI= 50 (Low); GL= 2.1 (Low); Net carb= 4.1 g

Beef—Liver: Braised, Broiled or Baked ☛ Serving size= 3 oz, 85 g; GI= 50 (Low); GL= 2.1 (Low); Net carb= 4.1 g

Beef—Liver: Fried, Stewed or Roast ☛ Serving size= 3 oz, 85 g; GI= 50 (Low); GL= 2.1 (Low); Net carb= 4.1 g

Beef—Loin Steaks and/or Steak Types ☛ Serving size= 3 oz, 85 g; GI= 0 (Low); GL= 0 (Low); Net carb= 0 g

Beef—Loin Steaks and/or Steak Types: Battered + fried ☛ Serving size= 3 oz, 85 g; GI= 0 (Low); GL= 0 (Low); Net carb= 17 g

Beef—Loin Steaks and/or Steak Types: Braised, Broiled or Baked ☛ Serving size= 3 oz, 85 g; GI= 0 (Low); GL= 0 (Low); Net carb= 0 g

Beef—Loin Steaks and/or Steak Types: Fried, Stewed or Roast ☛ Serving size= 3 oz, 85 g; GI= 0 (Low); GL= 0 (Low); Net carb= 0 g

Beef—Mock Tender Petite Fillet ☛ Serving size= 3 oz, 85 g; GI= 0 (Low); GL= 0 (Low); Net carb= 0 g

Beef—Mock Tender Petite Fillet: Battered + fried ☛ Serving size= 3 oz, 85 g; GI= 0 (Low); GL= 0 (Low); Net carb= 17 g

Beef—Mock Tender Petite Fillet: Braised, Broiled or Baked ☛ Serving size= 3 oz, 85 g; GI= 0 (Low); GL= 0 (Low); Net carb= 0 g

Beef—Mock Tender Petite Fillet: Fried, Stewed or Roast ☛ Serving size= 3 oz, 85 g; GI= 0 (Low); GL= 0 (Low); Net carb= 0 g

Beef—Prime Rib ☛ Serving size= 3 oz, 85 g; GI= 0 (Low); GL= 0 (Low); Net carb= 0 g

Beef—Prime Rib: Battered + fried ☛ Serving size= 3 oz, 85 g; GI= 0 (Low); GL= 0 (Low); Net carb= 17 g

Beef—Prime Rib: Braised, Broiled or Baked ☛ Serving size= 3 oz, 85 g; GI= 0 (Low); GL= 0 (Low); Net carb= 0 g

Beef—Prime Rib: Fried, Stewed or Roast ☛ Serving size= 3 oz, 85 g; GI= 0 (Low); GL= 0 (Low); Net carb= 0 g

Beef—Rib Steak Cuts ☛ Serving size= 3 oz, 85 g; GI= 0 (Low); GL= 0 (Low); Net carb= 0 g

Beef—Rib Steak Cuts: Battered + fried ☛ Serving size= 3 oz, 85 g; GI= 0 (Low); GL= 0 (Low); Net carb= 17 g

Beef—Rib Steak Cuts: Braised, Broiled or Baked ☛ Serving size= 3 oz, 85 g; GI= 0 (Low); GL= 0 (Low); Net carb= 0 g

Beef—Rib Steak Cuts: Fried, Stewed or Roast ☛ Serving size= 3 oz, 85 g; GI= 0 (Low); GL= 0 (Low); Net carb= 0 g

Beef—Round Steak Varieties ☛ Serving size= 3 oz, 85 g; GI= 0 (Low); GL= 0 (Low); Net carb= 0 g

Beef—Round Steak Varieties: Battered + fried ☛ Serving size= 3 oz, 85 g; GI= 0 (Low); GL= 0 (Low); Net carb= 17 g

Beef—Round Steak Varieties: Braised, Broiled or Baked ☛ Serving size= 3 oz, 85 g; GI= 0 (Low); GL= 0 (Low); Net carb= 0 g

Beef—Round Steak Varieties: Fried, Stewed or Roast ☛ Serving size= 3 oz, 85 g; GI= 0 (Low); GL= 0 (Low); Net carb= 0 g

Beef—Short Loin ☛ Serving size= 3 oz, 85 g; GI= 0 (Low); GL= 0 (Low); Net carb= 0 g

Beef—Short Loin: Battered + fried ☛ Serving size= 3 oz, 85 g; GI= 0 (Low); GL= 0 (Low); Net carb= 17 g

Beef—Short Loin: Braised, Broiled or Baked ☛ Serving size= 3 oz, 85 g; GI= 0 (Low); GL= 0 (Low); Net carb= 0 g

Beef—Short Loin: Fried, Stewed or Roast ☛ Serving size= 3 oz, 85 g; GI= 0 (Low); GL= 0 (Low); Net carb= 0 g

Beef—Short Ribs ☛ Serving size= 3 oz, 85 g; GI= 0 (Low); GL= 0 (Low); Net carb= 0 g

Beef—Short Ribs: Battered + fried ☛ Serving size= 3 oz, 85 g; GI= 0 (Low); GL= 0 (Low); Net carb= 17 g

Beef—Short Ribs: Braised, Broiled or Baked ☛ Serving size= 3 oz, 85 g; GI= 0 (Low); GL= 0 (Low); Net carb= 0 g

Beef—Short Ribs: Fried, Stewed or Roast ☛ Serving size= 3 oz, 85 g; GI= 0 (Low); GL= 0 (Low); Net carb= 0 g

Beef—T-Bone Steak ☛ Serving size= 3 oz, 85 g; GI= 0 (Low); GL= 0 (Low); Net carb= 0 g

Beef—T-Bone Steak: Battered + fried ☛ Serving size= 3 oz, 85 g; GI= 0 (Low); GL= 0 (Low); Net carb= 17 g

Beef—T-Bone Steak: Braised, Broiled or Baked ☛ Serving size= 3 oz, 85 g; GI= 0 (Low); GL= 0 (Low); Net carb= 0 g

Beef—T-Bone Steak: Fried, Stewed or Roast ☛ Serving size= 3 oz, 85 g; GI= 0 (Low); GL= 0 (Low); Net carb= 0 g

Beef—Tenderloin ☛ Serving size= 3 oz, 85 g; GI= 0 (Low); GL= 0 (Low); Net carb= 0 g

Beef—Tenderloin: Battered + fried ☛ Serving size= 3 oz, 85 g; GI= 0 (Low); GL= 0 (Low); Net carb= 17 g

Beef—Tenderloin: Braised, Broiled or Baked ☛ Serving size= 3 oz, 85 g; GI= 0 (Low); GL= 0 (Low); Net carb= 0 g

Beef—Tenderloin: Fried, Stewed or Roast ☛ Serving size= 3 oz, 85 g; GI= 0 (Low); GL= 0 (Low); Net carb= 0 g

Beef—Tongue ☛ Serving size= 3 oz, 85 g; GI= 0 (Low); GL= 0 (Low); Net carb= 0 g

Beef—Tongue: Braised, Broiled or Baked ☛ Serving size= 3 oz, 85 g; GI= 0 (Low); GL= 0 (Low); Net carb= 0 g

Beef—Tongue: Fried, Stewed or Roast ☛ Serving size= 3 oz, 85 g; GI= 0 (Low); GL= 0 (Low); Net carb= 0 g

Beef—Top Sirloin ☛ Serving size= 3 oz, 85 g; GI= 0 (Low); GL= 0 (Low); Net carb= 0 g

Beef—Top Sirloin: Battered + fried ☛ Serving size= 3 oz, 85 g; GI= 0 (Low); GL= 0 (Low); Net carb= 17 g

Beef—Top Sirloin: Braised, Broiled or Baked ☛ Serving size= 3 oz, 85 g; GI= 0 (Low); GL= 0 (Low); Net carb= 0 g

Beef—Top Sirloin: Fried, Stewed or Roast ☛ Serving size= 3 oz, 85 g; GI= 0 (Low); GL= 0 (Low); Net carb= 0 g

Beef—Tri-Tip ☛ Serving size= 3 oz, 85 g; GI= 0 (Low); GL= 0 (Low); Net carb= 0 g

Beef—Tri-Tip: Battered + fried ☛ Serving size= 3 oz, 85 g; GI= 0 (Low); GL= 0 (Low); Net carb= 17 g

Beef—Tri-Tip: Braised, Broiled or Baked ☛ Serving size= 3 oz, 85 g; GI= 0 (Low); GL= 0 (Low); Net carb= 0 g

Beef—Tri-Tip: Fried, Stewed or Roast ☛ Serving size= 3 oz, 85 g; GI= 0 (Low); GL= 0 (Low); Net carb= 0 g

Beef—Tripe ☛ Serving size= 3 oz, 85 g; GI= 0 (Low); GL= 0 (Low); Net carb= 0 g

Beef—Tripe: Braised, Broiled or Baked ☛ Serving size= 3 oz, 85 g; GI= 0 (Low); GL= 0 (Low); Net carb= 0 g

Beef—Tripe: Fried, Stewed or Roast ☛ Serving size= 3 oz, 85 g; GI= 0 (Low); GL= 0 (Low); Net carb= 0 g

Chicken—Backs and Necks ☛ Serving size= 3 oz, 85 g; GI= 0 (Low); GL= 0 (Low); Net carb= 0 g

Chicken—Backs and Necks: Braised, Broiled or Baked ☛ Serving size= 3 oz, 85 g; GI= 0 (Low); GL= 0 (Low); Net carb= 0 g

Chicken—Backs and Necks: Fried, Stewed or Roast ☛ Serving size= 3 oz, 85 g; GI= 0 (Low); GL= 0 (Low); Net carb= 0 g

Chicken—Breast Fillet Tenderloin ☛ Serving size= 3 oz, 85 g; GI= 0 (Low); GL= 0 (Low); Net carb= 0 g

Chicken—Breast Fillet Tenderloin: Braised, Broiled or Baked ☛ Serving size= 3 oz, 85 g; GI= 0 (Low); GL= 0 (Low); Net carb= 0 g

Chicken—Breast Fillet Tenderloin: Fried, Stewed or Roast ☛ Serving size= 3 oz, 85 g; GI= 0 (Low); GL= 0 (Low); Net carb= 0 g

Chicken—Drumstick ☛ Serving size= 3 oz, 85 g; GI= 0 (Low); GL= 0 (Low); Net carb= 0 g

Chicken—Drumstick: Braised, Broiled or Baked ☛ Serving size= 3 oz, 85 g; GI= 0 (Low); GL= 0 (Low); Net carb= 0 g

Chicken—Drumstick: Fried, Stewed or Roast ☛ Serving size= 3 oz, 85 g; GI= 0 (Low); GL= 0 (Low); Net carb= 0 g

Chicken—Leg ☛ Serving size= 3 oz, 85 g; GI= 0 (Low); GL= 0 (Low); Net carb= 0 g

Chicken—Leg: Braised, Broiled or Baked ☛ Serving size= 3 oz, 85 g; GI= 0 (Low); GL= 0 (Low); Net carb= 0 g

Chicken—Leg: Fried, Stewed or Roast ☛ Serving size= 3 oz, 85 g; GI= 0 (Low); GL= 0 (Low); Net carb= 0 g

Chicken—Tender ☛ Serving size= 3 oz, 85 g; GI= 0 (Low); GL= 0 (Low); Net carb= 0 g

Chicken—Tender: Braised, Broiled or Baked ☛ Serving size= 3 oz, 85 g; GI= 0 (Low); GL= 0 (Low); Net carb= 0 g

Chicken—Tender: Fried, Stewed or Roast ☛ Serving size= 3 oz, 85 g; GI= 0 (Low); GL= 0 (Low); Net carb= 0 g

Chicken—Thigh ☛ Serving size= 3 oz, 85 g; GI= 0 (Low); GL= 0 (Low); Net carb= 0 g

Chicken—Thigh: Braised, Broiled or Baked ☛ Serving size= 3 oz, 85 g; GI= 0 (Low); GL= 0 (Low); Net carb= 0 g

Chicken—Thigh: Fried, Stewed or Roast ☛ Serving size= 3 oz, 85 g; GI= 0 (Low); GL= 0 (Low); Net carb= 0 g

Chicken—Wing ☛ Serving size= 3 oz, 85 g; GI= 0 (Low); GL= 0 (Low); Net carb= 0 g

Chicken—Wing: Braised, Broiled or Baked ☛ Serving size= 3 oz, 85 g; GI= 0 (Low); GL= 0 (Low); Net carb= 0 g

Chicken—Wing: Fried, Stewed or Roast ☛ Serving size= 3 oz, 85 g; GI= 0 (Low); GL= 0 (Low); Net carb= 0 g

Eggs—Free-Range ☛ Serving size= 1 egg, 50 g; GI= (Low); GL= 0 (Low); Net carb= 0 g

Eggs—Free-Run ☛ Serving size= 1 egg, 50 g; GI= (Low); GL= 0 (Low); Net carb= 0 g

Eggs—Organic ☛ Serving size= 1 egg, 50 g; GI= (Low); GL= 0 (Low); Net carb= 0 g

Lamb—Breast ☛ Serving size= 3 oz, 85 g; GI= 0 (Low); GL= 0 (Low); Net carb= 0 g

Lamb—Breast: Braised, Broiled or Baked ☛ Serving size= 3 oz, 85 g; GI= 0 (Low); GL= 0 (Low); Net carb= 0 g

Lamb—Breast: Fried, Stewed or Roast ☛ Serving size= 3 oz, 85 g; GI= 0 (Low); GL= 0 (Low); Net carb= 0 g

Lamb—Cutlets ☛ Serving size= 3 oz, 85 g; GI= 0 (Low); GL= 0 (Low); Net carb= 0 g

Lamb—Cutlets: Braised, Broiled or Baked ☛ Serving size= 3 oz, 85 g; GI= 0 (Low); GL= 0 (Low); Net carb= 0 g

Lamb—Cutlets: Fried, Stewed or Roast ☛ Serving size= 3 oz, 85 g; GI= 0 (Low); GL= 0 (Low); Net carb= 0 g

Lamb—Leg ☛ Serving size= 3 oz, 85 g; GI= 0 (Low); GL= 0 (Low); Net carb= 0 g

Lamb—Leg: Braised, Broiled or Baked ☛ Serving size= 3 oz, 85 g; GI= 0 (Low); GL= 0 (Low); Net carb= 0 g

Lamb—Leg: Fried, Stewed or Roast ☛ Serving size= 3 oz, 85 g; GI= 0 (Low); GL= 0 (Low); Net carb= 0 g

Lamb—Loin ☛ Serving size= 3 oz, 85 g; GI= 0 (Low); GL= 0 (Low); Net carb= 0 g

Lamb—Loin: Braised, Broiled or Baked ☛ Serving size= 3 oz, 85 g; GI= 0 (Low); GL= 0 (Low); Net carb= 0 g

Lamb—Loin: Fried, Stewed or Roast ☛ Serving size= 3 oz, 85 g; GI= 0 (Low); GL= 0 (Low); Net carb= 0 g

Lamb—Neck ☛ Serving size= 3 oz, 85 g; GI= 0 (Low); GL= 0 (Low); Net carb= 0 g

Lamb—Neck: Braised, Broiled or Baked ☛ Serving size= 3 oz, 85 g; GI= 0 (Low); GL= 0 (Low); Net carb= 0 g

Lamb—Neck: Fried, Stewed or Roast ☛ Serving size= 3 oz, 85 g; GI= 0 (Low); GL= 0 (Low); Net carb= 0 g

Lamb—Rack ☛ Serving size= 3 oz, 85 g; GI= 0 (Low); GL= 0 (Low); Net carb= 0 g

Lamb—Rack: Braised, Broiled or Baked ☛ Serving size= 3 oz, 85 g; GI= 0 (Low); GL= 0 (Low); Net carb= 0 g

Lamb—Rack: Fried, Stewed or Roast ☛ Serving size= 3 oz, 85 g; GI= 0 (Low); GL= 0 (Low); Net carb= 0 g

Lamb—Rump ☛ Serving size= 3 oz, 85 g; GI= 0 (Low); GL= 0 (Low); Net carb= 0 g

Lamb—Rump: Braised, Broiled or Baked ☛ Serving size= 3 oz, 85 g; GI= 0 (Low); GL= 0 (Low); Net carb= 0 g

Lamb—Rump: Fried, Stewed or Roast ☛ Serving size= 3 oz, 85 g; GI= 0 (Low); GL= 0 (Low); Net carb= 0 g

Lamb—Shank ☛ Serving size= 3 oz, 85 g; GI= 0 (Low); GL= 0 (Low); Net carb= 0 g

Lamb—Shank: Braised, Broiled or Baked ☛ Serving size= 3 oz, 85 g; GI= 0 (Low); GL= 0 (Low); Net carb= 0 g

Lamb—Shank: Fried, Stewed or Roast ☛ Serving size= 3 oz, 85 g; GI= 0 (Low); GL= 0 (Low); Net carb= 0 g

Lamb—Shoulder ☛ Serving size= 3 oz, 85 g; GI= 0 (Low); GL= 0 (Low); Net carb= 0 g

Lamb—Shoulder: Braised, Broiled or Baked ☛ Serving size= 3 oz, 85 g; GI= 0 (Low); GL= 0 (Low); Net carb= 0 g

Lamb—Shoulder: Fried, Stewed or Roast ☛ Serving size= 3 oz, 85 g; GI= 0 (Low); GL= 0 (Low); Net carb= 0 g

Pork—back ribs ☛ Serving size= 3 oz, 85 g; GI= 0 (Low); GL= 0 (Low); Net carb= 0 g

Pork—back ribs: Braised, Broiled or Baked ☛ Serving size= 3 oz, 85 g; GI= 0 (Low); GL= 0 (Low); Net carb= 0 g

Pork—back ribs: Fried, Stewed or Roast ☛ Serving size= 3 oz, 85 g; GI= 0 (Low); GL= 0 (Low); Net carb= 0 g

Pork—Belly ☛ Serving size= 3 oz, 85 g; GI= 0 (Low); GL= 0 (Low); Net carb= 0 g

Pork—Belly: Braised, Broiled or Baked ☛ Serving size= 3 oz, 85 g; GI= 0 (Low); GL= 0 (Low); Net carb= 0 g

Pork—Belly: Fried, Stewed or Roast ☛ Serving size= 3 oz, 85 g; GI= 0 (Low); GL= 0 (Low); Net carb= 0 g

Pork—Cutlets ☛ Serving size= 3 oz, 85 g; GI= 0 (Low); GL= 0 (Low); Net carb= 0 g

Pork—Cutlets: Braised, Broiled or Baked ☛ Serving size= 3 oz, 85 g; GI= 0 (Low); GL= 0 (Low); Net carb= 0 g

Pork—Cutlets: Fried, Stewed or Roast ☛ Serving size= 3 oz, 85 g; GI= 0 (Low); GL= 0 (Low); Net carb= 0 g

Pork—Garlic Sausages ☛ Serving size= 3 oz, 85 g; GI= 0 (Low); GL= 0 (Low); Net carb= 0 g

Pork—Garlic Sausages: Braised, Broiled or Baked ☛ Serving size= 3 oz, 85 g; GI= 0 (Low); GL= 0 (Low); Net carb= 0 g

Pork—Garlic Sausages: Fried, Stewed or Roast ☛ Serving size= 3 oz, 85 g; GI= 0 (Low); GL= 0 (Low); Net carb= 0 g

Pork—Ham ☛ Serving size= 3 oz, 85 g; GI= 0 (Low); GL= 0 (Low); Net carb= 0 g

Pork—Ham: Braised, Broiled or Baked ☛ Serving size= 3 oz, 85 g; GI= 0 (Low); GL= 0 (Low); Net carb= 0 g

Pork—Ham: Fried, Stewed or Roast ☛ Serving size= 3 oz, 85 g; GI= 0 (Low); GL= 0 (Low); Net carb= 0 g

Pork—Loin ☛ Serving size= 3 oz, 85 g; GI= 0 (Low); GL= 0 (Low); Net carb= 0 g

Pork—Loin: Braised, Broiled or Baked ☛ Serving size= 3 oz, 85 g; GI= 0 (Low); GL= 0 (Low); Net carb= 0 g

Pork—Loin: Fried, Stewed or Roast ☛ Serving size= 3 oz, 85 g; GI= 0 (Low); GL= 0 (Low); Net carb= 0 g

Pork—Rib chops ☛ Serving size= 3 oz, 85 g; GI= 0 (Low); GL= 0 (Low); Net carb= 0 g

Pork—Rib chops: Braised, Broiled or Baked ☛ Serving size= 3 oz, 85 g; GI= 0 (Low); GL= 0 (Low); Net carb= 0 g

Pork—Rib chops: Fried, Stewed or Roast ☛ Serving size= 3 oz, 85 g; GI= 0 (Low); GL= 0 (Low); Net carb= 0 g

Pork—Roasts ☛ Serving size= 3 oz, 85 g; GI= 0 (Low); GL= 0 (Low); Net carb= 0 g

Pork—Roasts: Braised, Broiled or Baked ☛ Serving size= 3 oz, 85 g; GI= 0 (Low); GL= 0 (Low); Net carb= 0 g

Pork—Roasts: Fried, Stewed or Roast ☛ Serving size= 3 oz, 85 g; GI= 0 (Low); GL= 0 (Low); Net carb= 0 g

Pork—Sausages ☛ Serving size= 3 oz, 85 g; GI= 0 (Low); GL= 0 (Low); Net carb= 0 g

Pork—Sausages: Braised, Broiled or Baked ☛ Serving size= 3 oz, 85 g; GI= 0 (Low); GL= 0 (Low); Net carb= 0 g

Pork—Sausages: Fried, Stewed or Roast ☛ Serving size= 3 oz, 85 g; GI= 0 (Low); GL= 0 (Low); Net carb= 0 g

Pork—Shoulder chops ☛ Serving size= 3 oz, 85 g; GI= 0 (Low); GL= 0 (Low); Net carb= 0 g

Pork—Shoulder chops: Braised, Broiled or Baked ☛ Serving size= 3 oz, 85 g; GI= 0 (Low); GL= 0 (Low); Net carb= 0 g

Pork—Shoulder chops: Fried, Stewed or Roast ☛ Serving size= 3 oz, 85 g; GI= 0 (Low); GL= 0 (Low); Net carb= 0 g

Pork—Sirloin chops ☛ Serving size= 3 oz, 85 g; GI= 0 (Low); GL= 0 (Low); Net carb= 0 g

Pork—Sirloin chops: Braised, Broiled or Baked ☛ Serving size= 3 oz, 85 g; GI= 0 (Low); GL= 0 (Low); Net carb= 0 g

Pork—Sirloin chops: Fried, Stewed or Roast ☛ Serving size= 3 oz, 85 g; GI= 0 (Low); GL= 0 (Low); Net carb= 0 g

Pork—spare ribs ☛ Serving size= 3 oz, 85 g; GI= 0 (Low); GL= 0 (Low); Net carb= 0 g

Pork—spare ribs: Braised, Broiled or Baked ☛ Serving size= 3 oz, 85 g; GI= 0 (Low); GL= 0 (Low); Net carb= 0 g

Pork—spare ribs: Fried, Stewed or Roast ☛ Serving size= 3 oz, 85 g; GI= 0 (Low); GL= 0 (Low); Net carb= 0 g

Turkey—Backs and Necks ☛ Serving size= 3 oz, 85 g; GI= 0 (Low); GL= 0 (Low); Net carb= 0 g

Turkey—Backs and Necks: Braised, Broiled or Baked ☛ Serving size= 3 oz, 85 g; GI= 0 (Low); GL= 0 (Low); Net carb= 0 g

Turkey—Backs and Necks: Fried, Stewed or Roast ☛ Serving size= 3 oz, 85 g; GI= 0 (Low); GL= 0 (Low); Net carb= 0 g

Turkey—Breast ☛ Serving size= 3 oz, 85 g; GI= 0 (Low); GL= 0 (Low); Net carb= 0 g

Turkey—Breast Fillet Tenderloin ☛ Serving size= 3 oz, 85 g; GI= 0 (Low); GL= 0 (Low); Net carb= 0 g

Turkey—Breast Fillet Tenderloin: Braised, Broiled or Baked ☛ Serving size= 3 oz, 85 g; GI= 0 (Low); GL= 0 (Low); Net carb= 0 g

Turkey—Breast Fillet Tenderloin: Fried, Stewed or Roast ☛ Serving size= 3 oz, 85 g; GI= 0 (Low); GL= 0 (Low); Net carb= 0 g

Turkey—Breast: Braised, Broiled or Baked ☛ Serving size= 3 oz, 85 g; GI= 0 (Low); GL= 0 (Low); Net carb= 0 g

Turkey—Breast: Fried, Stewed or Roast ☛ Serving size= 3 oz, 85 g; GI= 0 (Low); GL= 0 (Low); Net carb= 0 g

Turkey—Drumstick ☛ Serving size= 3 oz, 85 g; GI= 0 (Low); GL= 0 (Low); Net carb= 0 g

Turkey—Drumstick: Braised, Broiled or Baked ☛ Serving size= 3 oz, 85 g; GI= 0 (Low); GL= 0 (Low); Net carb= 0 g

Turkey—Drumstick: Fried, Stewed or Roast ☛ Serving size= 3 oz, 85 g; GI= 0 (Low); GL= 0 (Low); Net carb= 0 g

Turkey—Leg ☛ Serving size= 3 oz, 85 g; GI= 0 (Low); GL= 0 (Low); Net carb= 0 g

Turkey—Leg: Braised, Broiled or Baked ☛ Serving size= 3 oz, 85 g; GI= 0 (Low); GL= 0 (Low); Net carb= 0 g

Turkey—Leg: Fried, Stewed or Roast ☛ Serving size= 3 oz, 85 g; GI= 0 (Low); GL= 0 (Low); Net carb= 0 g

Turkey—Tender ☛ Serving size= 3 oz, 85 g; GI= 0 (Low); GL= 0 (Low); Net carb= 0 g

Turkey—Tender: Braised, Broiled or Baked ☛ Serving size= 3 oz, 85 g; GI= 0 (Low); GL= 0 (Low); Net carb= 0 g

Turkey—Tender: Fried, Stewed or Roast ☛ Serving size= 3 oz, 85 g; GI= 0 (Low); GL= 0 (Low); Net carb= 0 g

Turkey—Thigh ☛ Serving size= 3 oz, 85 g; GI= 0 (Low); GL= 0 (Low); Net carb= 0 g

Turkey—Thigh: Braised, Broiled or Baked ☛ Serving size= 3 oz, 85 g; GI= 0 (Low); GL= 0 (Low); Net carb= 0 g

Turkey—Thigh: Fried, Stewed or Roast ☛ Serving size= 3 oz, 85 g; GI= 0 (Low); GL= 0 (Low); Net carb= 0 g

Turkey—Wing ☛ Serving size= 3 oz, 85 g; GI= 0 (Low); GL= 0 (Low); Net carb= 0 g

Turkey—Wing: Braised, Broiled or Baked ☛ Serving size= 3 oz, 85 g; GI= 0 (Low); GL= 0 (Low); Net carb= 0 g

Turkey—Wing: Fried, Stewed or Roast ☛ Serving size= 3 oz, 85 g; GI= 0 (Low); GL= 0 (Low); Net carb= 0 g

Veal-Offal—Heart ☛ Serving size= 3 oz, 85 g; GI= 0 (Low); GL= 0 (Low); Net carb= 0 g

Veal-Offal—Heart: Braised, Broiled or Baked ☛ Serving size= 3 oz, 85 g; GI= 0 (Low); GL= 0 (Low); Net carb= 0 g

Veal-Offal—Heart: Fried, Stewed or Roast ☛ Serving size= 3 oz, 85 g; GI= 0 (Low); GL= 0 (Low); Net carb= 0 g

Veal—Bottom Round ☛ Serving size= 3 oz, 85 g; GI= 0 (Low); GL= 0 (Low); Net carb= 0 g

Veal—Bottom Round: Braised, Broiled or Baked ☛ Serving size= 3 oz, 85 g; GI= 0 (Low); GL= 0 (Low); Net carb= 0 g

Veal—Bottom Round: Fried, Stewed or Roast ☛ Serving size= 3 oz, 85 g; GI= 0 (Low); GL= 0 (Low); Net carb= 0 g

Veal—Brain ☛ Serving size= 3 oz, 85 g; GI= 0 (Low); GL= 0 (Low); Net carb= 0 g

Veal—Brain: Braised, Broiled or Baked ☛ Serving size= 3 oz, 85 g; GI= 0 (Low); GL= 0 (Low); Net carb= 0 g

Veal—Brain: Fried, Stewed or Roast ☛ Serving size= 3 oz, 85 g; GI= 0 (Low); GL= 0 (Low); Net carb= 0 g

Veal—Brisket ☛ Serving size= 3 oz, 85 g; GI= 0 (Low); GL= 0 (Low); Net carb= 0 g

Veal—Brisket: Braised, Broiled or Baked ☛ Serving size= 3 oz, 85 g; GI= 0 (Low); GL= 0 (Low); Net carb= 0 g

Veal—Brisket: Fried, Stewed or Roast ☛ Serving size= 3 oz, 85 g; GI= 0 (Low); GL= 0 (Low); Net carb= 0 g

Veal—Chuck Roast ☛ Serving size= 3 oz, 85 g; GI= 0 (Low); GL= 0 (Low); Net carb= 0 g

Veal—Chuck Roast: Braised, Broiled or Baked ☛ Serving size= 3 oz, 85 g; GI= 0 (Low); GL= 0 (Low); Net carb= 0 g

Veal—Chuck Roast: Fried, Stewed or Roast ☛ Serving size= 3 oz, 85 g; GI= 0 (Low); GL= 0 (Low); Net carb= 0 g

Veal—Chuck Steak Varieties Chart ☛ Serving size= 3 oz, 85 g; GI= 0 (Low); GL= 0 (Low); Net carb= 0 g

Veal—Chuck Steak Varieties Chart: Braised, Broiled or Baked ☛ Serving size= 3 oz, 85 g; GI= 0 (Low); GL= 0 (Low); Net carb= 0 g

Veal—Chuck Steak Varieties Chart: Fried, Stewed or Roast ☛ Serving size= 3 oz, 85 g; GI= 0 (Low); GL= 0 (Low); Net carb= 0 g

Veal—Cuts of Steak ☛ Serving size= 3 oz, 85 g; GI= 0 (Low); GL= 0 (Low); Net carb= 0 g

Veal—Cuts of Steak: Braised, Broiled or Baked ☛ Serving size= 3 oz, 85 g; GI= 0 (Low); GL= 0 (Low); Net carb= 0 g

Veal—Cuts of Steak: Fried, Stewed or Roast ☛ Serving size= 3 oz, 85 g; GI= 0 (Low); GL= 0 (Low); Net carb= 0 g

Veal—Delmonico Steak ☛ Serving size= 3 oz, 85 g; GI= 0 (Low); GL= 0 (Low); Net carb= 0 g

Veal—Delmonico Steak: Braised, Broiled or Baked ☛ Serving size= 3 oz, 85 g; GI= 0 (Low); GL= 0 (Low); Net carb= 0 g

Veal—Delmonico Steak: Fried, Stewed or Roast ☛ Serving size= 3 oz, 85 g; GI= 0 (Low); GL= 0 (Low); Net carb= 0 g

Veal—Hanger Steak ☛ Serving size= 3 oz, 85 g; GI= 0 (Low); GL= 0 (Low); Net carb= 0 g

Veal—Hanger Steak: Braised, Broiled or Baked ☛ Serving size= 3 oz, 85 g; GI= 0 (Low); GL= 0 (Low); Net carb= 0 g

Veal—Hanger Steak: Fried, Stewed or Roast ☛ Serving size= 3 oz, 85 g; GI= 0 (Low); GL= 0 (Low); Net carb= 0 g

Veal—Kidney ☛ Serving size= 3 oz, 85 g; GI= 0 (Low); GL= 0 (Low); Net carb= 0 g

Veal—Kidney: Braised, Broiled or Baked ☛ Serving size= 3 oz, 85 g; GI= 0 (Low); GL= 0 (Low); Net carb= 0 g

Veal—Kidney: Fried, Stewed or Roast ☛ Serving size= 3 oz, 85 g; GI= 0 (Low); GL= 0 (Low); Net carb= 0 g

Veal—Liver ☛ Serving size= 1 slice, 81 g; GI= 50 (Low); GL= 2.1 (Low); Net carb= 4.1 g

Veal—Liver: Braised, Broiled or Baked ☛ Serving size= 1 slice, 81 g; GI= 50 (Low); GL= 2.1 (Low); Net carb= 4.1 g

Veal—Liver: Fried, Stewed or Roast ☛ Serving size= 1 slice, 81 g; GI= 50 (Low); GL= 2.1 (Low); Net carb= 4.1 g

Veal—Loin Steaks and/or Steak Types ☛ Serving size= 3 oz, 85 g; GI= 0 (Low); GL= 0 (Low); Net carb= 0 g

Veal—Loin Steaks and/or Steak Types: Braised, Broiled or Baked ☛ Serving size= 3 oz, 85 g; GI= 0 (Low); GL= 0 (Low); Net carb= 0 g

Veal—Loin Steaks and/or Steak Types: Fried, Stewed or Roast ☛ Serving size= 3 oz, 85 g; GI= 0 (Low); GL= 0 (Low); Net carb= 0 g

Veal—Mock Tender Petite Fillet ☛ Serving size= 3 oz, 85 g; GI= 0 (Low); GL= 0 (Low); Net carb= 0 g

Veal—Mock Tender Petite Fillet: Braised, Broiled or Baked ☛ Serving size= 3 oz, 85 g; GI= 0 (Low); GL= 0 (Low); Net carb= 0 g

Veal—Mock Tender Petite Fillet: Fried, Stewed or Roast ☛ Serving size= 3 oz, 85 g; GI= 0 (Low); GL= 0 (Low); Net carb= 0 g

Veal—Prime Rib ☛ Serving size= 3 oz, 85 g; GI= 0 (Low); GL= 0 (Low); Net carb= 0 g

Veal—Prime Rib: Braised, Broiled or Baked ☛ Serving size= 3 oz, 85 g; GI= 0 (Low); GL= 0 (Low); Net carb= 0 g

Veal—Prime Rib: Fried, Stewed or Roast ☛ Serving size= 3 oz, 85 g; GI= 0 (Low); GL= 0 (Low); Net carb= 0 g

Veal—Rib Steak Cuts ☛ Serving size= 3 oz, 85 g; GI= 0 (Low); GL= 0 (Low); Net carb= 0 g

Veal—Rib Steak Cuts: Braised, Broiled or Baked ☛ Serving size= 3 oz, 85 g; GI= 0 (Low); GL= 0 (Low); Net carb= 0 g

Veal—Rib Steak Cuts: Fried, Stewed or Roast ☛ Serving size= 3 oz, 85 g; GI= 0 (Low); GL= 0 (Low); Net carb= 0 g

Veal—Round Steak Varieties ☛ Serving size= 3 oz, 85 g; GI= 0 (Low); GL= 0 (Low); Net carb= 0 g

Veal—Round Steak Varieties: Braised, Broiled or Baked ☛ Serving size= 3 oz, 85 g; GI= 0 (Low); GL= 0 (Low); Net carb= 0 g

Veal—Round Steak Varieties: Fried, Stewed or Roast ☛ Serving size= 3 oz, 85 g; GI= 0 (Low); GL= 0 (Low); Net carb= 0 g

Veal—Short Loin ☛ Serving size= 3 oz, 85 g; GI= 0 (Low); GL= 0 (Low); Net carb= 0 g

Veal—Short Loin: Braised, Broiled or Baked ☛ Serving size= 3 oz, 85 g; GI= 0 (Low); GL= 0 (Low); Net carb= 0 g

Veal—Short Loin: Fried, Stewed or Roast ☛ Serving size= 3 oz, 85 g; GI= 0 (Low); GL= 0 (Low); Net carb= 0 g

Veal—Short Ribs ☛ Serving size= 3 oz, 85 g; GI= 0 (Low); GL= 0 (Low); Net carb= 0 g

Veal—Short Ribs: Braised, Broiled or Baked ☛ Serving size= 3 oz, 85 g; GI= 0 (Low); GL= 0 (Low); Net carb= 0 g

Veal—Short Ribs: Fried, Stewed or Roast ☛ Serving size= 3 oz, 85 g; GI= 0 (Low); GL= 0 (Low); Net carb= 0 g

Veal—T-Bone Steak ☛ Serving size= 3 oz, 85 g; GI= 0 (Low); GL= 0 (Low); Net carb= 0 g

Veal—T-Bone Steak: Braised, Broiled or Baked ☛ Serving size= 3 oz, 85 g; GI= 0 (Low); GL= 0 (Low); Net carb= 0 g

Veal—T-Bone Steak: Fried, Stewed or Roast ☛ Serving size= 3 oz, 85 g; GI= 0 (Low); GL= 0 (Low); Net carb= 0 g

Veal—Tenderloin ☛ Serving size= 3 oz, 85 g; GI= 0 (Low); GL= 0 (Low); Net carb= 0 g

Veal—Tenderloin: Braised, Broiled or Baked ☛ Serving size= 3 oz, 85 g; GI= 0 (Low); GL= 0 (Low); Net carb= 0 g

Veal—Tenderloin: Fried, Stewed or Roast ☛ Serving size= 3 oz, 85 g; GI= 0 (Low); GL= 0 (Low); Net carb= 0 g

Veal—Tongue ☛ Serving size= 3 oz, 85 g; GI= 0 (Low); GL= 0 (Low); Net carb= 0 g

Veal—Tongue: Braised, Broiled or Baked ☛ Serving size= 3 oz, 85 g; GI= 0 (Low); GL= 0 (Low); Net carb= 0 g

Veal—Tongue: Fried, Stewed or Roast ☛ Serving size= 3 oz, 85 g; GI= 0 (Low); GL= 0 (Low); Net carb= 0 g

Veal—Top Sirloin ☛ Serving size= 3 oz, 85 g; GI= 0 (Low); GL= 0 (Low); Net carb= 0 g

Veal—Top Sirloin: Braised, Broiled or Baked ☛ Serving size= 3 oz, 85 g; GI= 0 (Low); GL= 0 (Low); Net carb= 0 g

Veal—Top Sirloin: Fried, Stewed or Roast ☛ Serving size= 3 oz, 85 g; GI= 0 (Low); GL= 0 (Low); Net carb= 0 g

Veal—Tri-Tip ☛ Serving size= 3 oz, 85 g; GI= 0 (Low); GL= 0 (Low); Net carb= 0 g

Veal—Tri-Tip: Braised, Broiled or Baked ☛ Serving size= 3 oz, 85 g; GI= 0 (Low); GL= 0 (Low); Net carb= 0 g

Veal—Tri-Tip: Fried, Stewed or Roast ☛ Serving size= 3 oz, 85 g; GI= 0 (Low); GL= 0 (Low); Net carb= 0 g

Veal—Tripe ☛ Serving size= 3 oz, 85 g; GI= 0 (Low); GL= 0 (Low); Net carb= 0 g

Veal—Tripe: Braised, Broiled or Baked ☛ Serving size= 3 oz, 85 g; GI= 0 (Low); GL= 0 (Low); Net carb= 0 g

Veal—Tripe: Fried, Stewed or Roast ☛ Serving size= 3 oz, 85 g; GI= 0 (Low); GL= 0 (Low); Net carb= 0 g

28

BEVERAGES

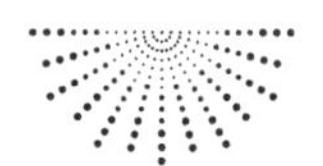

— People with diabetes should avoid heavy drinking

Acai Berry Drink Enriched ☛ Serving size= 8 fl oz, 266 g; GI= 27 (Low); GL= 8.4 (Low); Net carb= 30.9 g

Alcoholic Beverage—100 Proof Liquor ☛ Serving size= 1 fl oz, 27.8 g; GI= 0 (Low); GL= 0 (Low); Net carb= 0 g

Alcoholic Beverage—86 Proof Liquor ☛ Serving size= 1 fl oz, 27.8 g; GI= 0 (Low); GL= 0 (Low); Net carb= 0 g

Alcoholic Beverage—90 Proof Liquor ☛ Serving size= 1 fl oz, 27.8 g; GI= 0 (Low); GL= 0 (Low); Net carb= 0 g

Alcoholic Beverage—94 Proof Liquor ☛ Serving size= 1 fl oz, 27.8 g; GI= 0 (Low); GL= 0 (Low); Net carb= 0 g

Alcoholic Beverage—Beer ☛ Serving size= 1 fl oz, 29.7 g; GI= 100 (High); GL= 1.1 (Low); Net carb= 1.1 g

Alcoholic Beverage—Creme De Menthe 72 Proof ☛ Serving size= 1 fl oz, 33.6 g; GI= 63 (Medium); GL= 8.8 (Low); Net carb= 14 g

Alcoholic Beverage—Daiquiri Made-From-Recipe ☛ Serving size= 1 fl oz, 30.2 g; GI= 15 (Low); GL= 0.3 (Low); Net carb= 2.1 g

Alcoholic Beverage—Gin ☛ Serving size= 1 fl oz, 27.8 g; GI= 0 (Low); GL= 0 (Low); Net carb= 0 g

Alcoholic Beverage—Liqueur Coffee 63 Proof ☛ Serving size= 1 fl oz, 34.8 g; GI= 63 (Medium); GL= 7.1 (Low); Net carb= 11.2 g

Alcoholic Beverage—Muscat Wine ☛ Serving size= 1 fl oz, 30 g; GI= 7 (Low); GL= 0.1 (Low); Net carb= 1.6 g

Alcoholic Beverage—Pina Colada Canned ☛ Serving size= 1 fl oz, 32.6 g; GI= 35 (Low); GL= 3.1 (Low); Net carb= 9 g

Alcoholic Beverage—Pina Colada Made-From-Recipe ☛ Serving size= 1 fl oz, 31.4 g; GI= 15 (Low); GL= 1.1 (Low); Net carb= 7 g

Alcoholic Beverage—Red Wine ☛ Serving size= 1 fl oz, 29.4 g; GI= 7 (Low); GL= 0.1 (Low); Net carb= 0.8 g

Alcoholic Beverage—Rice (Sake) ☛ Serving size= 1 fl oz, 29.1 g; GI= 66 (Medium); GL= 1 (Low); Net carb= 1.5 g

Alcoholic Beverage—Rose Wine ☛ Serving size= 1 fl oz, 30.3 g; GI= 7 (Low); GL= 0.1 (Low); Net carb= 1.2 g

Alcoholic Beverage—Rum ☛ Serving size= 1 fl oz, 27.8 g; GI= 0 (Low); GL= 0 (Low); Net carb= 0 g

Alcoholic Beverage—Sauvignon Blanc ☛ Serving size= 1 fl oz, 29.3 g; GI= 7 (Low); GL= 0 (Low); Net carb= 0.6 g

Alcoholic Beverage—Semillon ☛ Serving size= 1 fl oz, 29.5 g; GI= 7 (Low); GL= 0.1 (Low); Net carb= 0.9 g

Alcoholic Beverage—Table Wine ☛ Serving size= 1 serving (5 fl oz), 148 g; GI= 7 (Low); GL= 0.3 (Low); Net carb= 4 g

Alcoholic Beverage—Vodka ☛ Serving size= 1 fl oz, 27.8 g; GI= 0 (Low); GL= 0 (Low); Net carb= 0 g

Alcoholic Beverage—Whiskey ☛ Serving size= 1 fl oz, 27.8 g; GI= 0 (Low); GL= 0 (Low); Net carb= 0 g

Alcoholic Beverage—Whiskey Sour ☛ Serving size= 1 fl oz, 30.4 g; GI= 73 (High); GL= 2.9 (Low); Net carb= 4 g

Alcoholic Beverage—Whiskey Sour Canned ☛ Serving size= 1 fl oz, 30.8 g; GI= 73 (High); GL= 3 (Low); Net carb= 4.1 g

Alcoholic Beverage—White Wine ☛ Serving size= 1 fl oz, 29.4 g; GI= 7 (Low); GL= 0.1 (Low); Net carb= 0.8 g

Alcoholic Beverage—Wine Cooking ☛ Serving size= 1 tsp, 4.9 g; GI= 11 (Low); GL= 0 (Low); Net carb= 0.3 g

Alcoholic Beverage—Wine Light ☛ Serving size= 1 fl oz, 29.5 g; GI= 7 (Low); GL= 0 (Low); Net carb= 0.3 g

Aloe Vera Juice Drink Enriched With Vitamin C ☛ Serving size= 8 fl oz, 240 g; GI= 66 (Medium); GL= 5.9 (Low); Net carb= 9 g

Apple Cider ☛ Serving size= 12 fl oz, 355 g; GI= 40 (Low); GL= 8.4 (Low); Net carb= 21 g

Barbera ☛ Serving size= 1 fl oz, 29.4 g; GI= 7 (Low); GL= 0.1 (Low); Net carb= 0.8 g

Bottled Water ☛ Serving size= 1 fl oz, 29.6 g; GI= 0 (Low); GL= 0 (Low); Net carb= 0 g

Cabernet Franc ☛ Serving size= 1 fl oz, 29.4 g; GI= 7 (Low); GL= 0.1 (Low); Net carb= 0.7 g

Cabernet Sauvignon ☛ Serving size= 1 fl oz, 29.4 g; GI= 7 (Low); GL= 0.1 (Low); Net carb= 0.8 g

Caffeine Free Cola ☛ Serving size= 1 fl oz, 30.7 g; GI= 65 (Medium); GL= 2.1 (Low); Net carb= 3.2 g

Carbonated Beverage—Low Calorie Other Than Cola Or Pepper With Sodium Saccharin Without Caffeine ☛ Serving size= 1 fl oz,

29.6 g; GI= 54 (Low); GL= 0 (Low); Net carb= 0 g

Carbonated Beverage—Other Than Cola Or Pepper, Low Calorie With Aspartame Contains Caffeine ☛ Serving size= 1 fl oz, 29.6 g; GI= 54 (Low); GL= 0 (Low); Net carb= 0 g

Carbonated Beverage—Other Than Cola Or Pepper, Low Calorie Without Caffeine ☛ Serving size= 1 fl oz, 29.6 g; GI= 54 (Low); GL= 0 (Low); Net carb= 0 g

Cereal Beverage ☛ Serving size= 1 fl oz, 30 g; GI= 7 (Low); GL= 0 (Low); Net carb= 0.2 g

Cereal Beverage—With Beet Roots From Powdered Instant ☛ Serving size= 1 fl oz, 30 g; GI= 7 (Low); GL= 0 (Low); Net carb= 0.2 g

Champagne Punch ☛ Serving size= 1 fl oz, 30 g; GI= 68 (Medium); GL= 2.5 (Low); Net carb= 3.6 g

Chardonnay ☛ Serving size= 1 fl oz, 29.3 g; GI= 7 (Low); GL= 0 (Low); Net carb= 0.6 g

Chenin Blanc ☛ Serving size= 1 fl oz, 29.5 g; GI= 7 (Low); GL= 0.1 (Low); Net carb= 1 g

Chicory Beverage ☛ Serving size= 1 fl oz, 30 g; GI= 9 (Low); GL= 0 (Low); Net carb= 0.4 g

Citrus Fruit Juice Drink—Frozen Concentrate ☛ Serving size= 1 fl oz, 35.2 g; GI= 69 (Medium); GL= 9.7 (Low); Net carb= 14.1 g

Citrus Fruit Juice Drink—Frozen—Concentrate—Made With Water ☛ Serving size= 1 fl oz, 31 g; GI= 59 (Medium); GL= 2.1 (Low); Net carb= 3.5 g

Citrus Green Tea ☛ Serving size= 1 cup, 265 g; GI= 0 (Low); GL= 0 (Low); Net carb= 0.8 g

Cocoa Mix Powder Made With Water ☛ Serving size= 1 fl oz, 34.3 g; GI= 77 (High); GL= 2.9 (Low); Net carb= 3.8 g

Cocoa Mix With Aspartame Powder Made With Water ☛ Serving size= 1 fl oz, 32.1 g; GI= 35 (Low); GL= 0.6 (Low); Net carb= 1.6 g

Coconut Milk Sweetened Enriched With Calcium Vitamins A B12 D2 ☛ Serving size= 1 cup, 240 g; GI= 41 (Low); GL= 2.9 (Low); Net carb= 7 g

Coconut Water—Ready-To-Drink—Unsweetened ☛ Serving size= 1 cup, 245 g; GI= 41 (Low); GL= 4.3 (Low); Net carb= 10.4 g

Coffee ☛ Serving size= 1 fl oz, 29.6 g; GI= 0 (Low); GL= 0 (Low); Net carb= 0 g

Coffee Instant—Chicory ☛ Serving size= 1 fl oz, 29.9 g; GI= 7 (Low); GL= 0 (Low); Net carb= 0.2 g

Coffee Instant—Chicory, Powder ☛ Serving size= 1 tsp, rounded, 1.8 g; GI= 89 (High); GL= 1.3 (Low); Net carb= 1.4 g

Coffee Instant—Decaffeinated Powder ☛ Serving size= 1 tsp rounded, 1.8 g; GI= 89 (High); GL= 1.2 (Low); Net carb= 1.4 g

Coffee Instant—Mocha Sweetened ☛ Serving size= 1 serving 2 tbsp, 13 g; GI= 89 (High); GL= 8.3 (Low); Net carb= 9.4 g

Coffee Instant—Reconstituted ☛ Serving size= 1 fl oz, 30 g; GI= 0 (Low); GL= 0 (Low); Net carb= 0.2 g

Coffee Instant—Regular Half The Caffeine ☛ Serving size= 1 tsp, 1 g; GI= 89 (High); GL= 0.7 (Low); Net carb= 0.7 g

Coffee Instant—Regular Powder ☛ Serving size= 1 tsp, 1 g; GI= 89 (High); GL= 0.7 (Low); Net carb= 0.8 g

Coffee Instant—With Whitener Reduced Calorie ☛ Serving size= 1 tsp dry, 1.7 g; GI= 77 (High); GL= 0.8 (Low); Net carb= 1 g

Coffee—Bottled or canned, Light ☛ Serving size= 1 fl oz, 30 g; GI= 21 (Low); GL= 0.4 (Low); Net carb= 1.8 g

Coffee—Brewed—Blend Of Regular And Decaffeinated ☛ Serving size= 1 fl oz, 30 g; GI= 0 (Low); GL= 0 (Low); Net carb= 0 g

Coffee—Brewed—Breakfast Blend ☛ Serving size= 1 cup, 248 g; GI= 0 (Low); GL= 0 (Low); Net carb= 0.4 g

Coffee—Brewed—Espresso Restaurant-Made Decaffeinated ☛ Serving size= 1 fl oz, 29.6 g; GI= 0 (Low); GL= 0 (Low); Net carb= 0.5 g

Coffee—Cafe Con Leche ☛ Serving size= 1 fl oz, 31 g; GI= 5 (Low); GL= 0.1 (Low); Net carb= 1.7 g

Coffee—Cafe Con Leche Decaffeinated ☛ Serving size= 1 fl oz, 31 g; GI= 21 (Low); GL= 0.4 (Low); Net carb= 1.8 g

Coffee—Cafe Mocha ☛ Serving size= 1 fl oz, 31 g; GI= 21 (Low); GL= 0.7 (Low); Net carb= 3.1 g

Coffee—Cappuccino ☛ Serving size= 1 fl oz, 30 g; GI= 33 (Low); GL= 0.3 (Low); Net carb= 0.8 g

Coffee—Cuban ☛ Serving size= 1 fl oz, 31 g; GI= 41 (Low); GL= 1 (Low); Net carb= 2.4 g

Coffee—Espresso ☛ Serving size= 1 fl oz, 29.6 g; GI= 0 (Low); GL= 0 (Low); Net carb= 0.5 g

Coffee—Latte ☛ Serving size= 1 fl oz, 30 g; GI= 21 (Low); GL= 0.3 (Low); Net carb= 1.3 g

Coffee—Macchiato ☛ Serving size= 1 fl oz, 30 g; GI= 21 (Low); GL= 0.2 (Low); Net carb= 0.8 g

Coffee—Turkish ☛ Serving size= 1 fl oz, 31 g; GI= 51 (Low); GL= 1 (Low); Net carb= 2 g

Cola Soft Drink ☛ Serving size= 1 fl oz, 30.7 g; GI= 69 (Medium); GL= 2.2 (Low); Net carb= 3.2 g

Corn Beverage ☛ Serving size= 1 fl oz, 30 g; GI= 55 (Medium); GL=

1.5 (Low); Net carb= 2.7 g

Cornmeal Beverage ☛ Serving size= 1 cup, 248 g; GI= (); GL= 0 (Low); Net carb= 40.2 g

Cranberry Juice Cocktail Bottled ☛ Serving size= 1 fl oz, 31.6 g; GI= 59 (Medium); GL= 2.5 (Low); Net carb= 4.3 g

Cranberry Juice Cocktail Frozen—Concentrate—Made With Water ☛ Serving size= 1 fl oz, 29.6 g; GI= 59 (Medium); GL= 2.1 (Low); Net carb= 3.5 g

Diet Cola ☛ Serving size= 1 fl oz, 29.6 g; GI= 41 (Low); GL= 0.6 (Low); Net carb= 1.5 g

Diet Green Tea ☛ Serving size= 1 cup, 269 g; GI= 11 (Low); GL= 0.3 (Low); Net carb= 2.5 g

Diet Pepper Cola ☛ Serving size= 1 fl oz, 29.6 g; GI= 11 (Low); GL= 0 (Low); Net carb= 0 g

Energy Drink Amp Sugar Free ☛ Serving size= 8 fl oz, 240 g; GI= 0 (Low); GL= 0 (Low); Net carb= 2.5 g

Energy Drink—Low Carb Monster ☛ Serving size= 8 fl oz, 240 g; GI= 15 (Low); GL= 0.5 (Low); Net carb= 3.3 g

Energy Drink—Rockstar ☛ Serving size= 1 fl oz, 31 g; GI= 68 (Medium); GL= 2.7 (Low); Net carb= 3.9 g

Energy Drink—Rockstar Sugar Free ☛ Serving size= 8 fl oz, 240 g; GI= 0 (Low); GL= 0 (Low); Net carb= 1.7 g

Energy Drink—Sugar Free ☛ Serving size= 8 fl oz, 240 g; GI= 0 (Low); GL= 0 (Low); Net carb= 1 g

Energy Drink—Vault Citrus Flavor ☛ Serving size= 1 oz, 31 g; GI= 68 (Medium); GL= 2.7 (Low); Net carb= 4 g

Energy Drink—Vault Zero Sugar-Free Citrus Flavor ☛ Serving size= 1 serving (8 fl oz), 246 g; GI= 0 (Low); GL= 0 (Low); Net carb= 1.7 g

Fluid Replacement 5% Glucose In Water ☛ Serving size= 1 cup, 240 g; GI= 40 (Low); GL= 4.8 (Low); Net carb= 12 g

Frozen Coffee—Drink ☛ Serving size= 1 fl oz, 31 g; GI= 55 (Medium); GL= 2.3 (Low); Net carb= 4.2 g

Frozen Coffee—Drink Decaffeinated ☛ Serving size= 1 fl oz, 31 g; GI= 55 (Medium); GL= 2.3 (Low); Net carb= 4.2 g

Frozen Coffee—Drink Decaffeinated Nonfat ☛ Serving size= 1 fl oz, 31 g; GI= 55 (Medium); GL= 2.3 (Low); Net carb= 4.2 g

Frozen Coffee—Drink Nonfat ☛ Serving size= 1 fl oz, 31 g; GI= 55 (Medium); GL= 2.3 (Low); Net carb= 4.2 g

Frozen Coffee—Drink Nonfat With Whipped Cream ☛ Serving size= 1 fl oz, 31 g; GI= 55 (Medium); GL= 2.2 (Low); Net carb= 4 g

Frozen Coffee—Drink With Non-Dairy Milk ☛ Serving size= 1 fl oz, 31 g; GI= 55 (Medium); GL= 2.3 (Low); Net carb= 4.3 g

Fruit And Vegetable Smoothie ☛ Serving size= 1 fl oz, 27 g; GI= 55 (Medium); GL= 1.8 (Low); Net carb= 3.2 g

Fruit And Vegetable Smoothie Added Protein ☛ Serving size= 1 fl oz, 27 g; GI= 55 (Medium); GL= 1.7 (Low); Net carb= 3 g

Fruit Flavored Drink With High Vitamin C Powdered Reconstituted ☛ Serving size= 1 fl oz (no ice), 31 g; GI= 68 (Medium); GL= 2.2 (Low); Net carb= 3.2 g

Fruit Flavored Smoothie Drink Frozen Light No Dairy ☛ Serving size= 1 fl oz, 30 g; GI= 68 (Medium); GL= 0.7 (Low); Net carb= 1 g

Fruit Flavored Smoothie Drink Frozen No Dairy ☛ Serving size= 1 fl oz, 30 g; GI= 68 (Medium); GL= 1.6 (Low); Net carb= 2.3 g

Fruit Juice Drink—Citrus Carbonated ☛ Serving size= 1 fl oz (no ice), 31 g; GI= 68 (Medium); GL= 1.4 (Low); Net carb= 2 g

Fruit Juice Drink—Diet ☛ Serving size= 1 fl oz (no ice), 30 g; GI= 0

(Low); GL= 0 (Low); Net carb= 0.1 g

Fruit Juice Drink—Noncitrus Carbonated ☛ Serving size= 1 fl oz (no ice), 31 g; GI= 68 (Medium); GL= 1.7 (Low); Net carb= 2.6 g

Fruit Juice Drink—Reduced Sugar (Sunny D) ☛ Serving size= 1 fl oz (no ice), 31 g; GI= 0 (Low); GL= 0 (Low); Net carb= 0.3 g

Fruit Smoothie (average value) ☛ Serving size= 1 fl oz, 27 g; GI= 77 (High); GL= 2.2 (Low); Net carb= 2.8 g

Fruit Smoothie—Light ☛ Serving size= 1 fl oz, 27 g; GI= 77 (High); GL= 1.8 (Low); Net carb= 2.3 g

Fruit Smoothie—With Whole Fruit And Dairy ☛ Serving size= 1 fl oz, 27 g; GI= 77 (High); GL= 2.2 (Low); Net carb= 2.8 g

Fruit Smoothie—With Whole Fruit And Dairy Added Protein ☛ Serving size= 1 fl oz, 27 g; GI= 77 (High); GL= 1.8 (Low); Net carb= 2.3 g

Fruit Smoothie—With Whole Fruit No Dairy ☛ Serving size= 1 fl oz, 27 g; GI= 77 (High); GL= 2.4 (Low); Net carb= 3.1 g

Fruit Smoothie—With Whole Fruit No Dairy Added Protein ☛ Serving size= 1 fl oz, 27 g; GI= 77 (High); GL= 2.2 (Low); Net carb= 2.9 g

Fruit-Flavored Drink—Dry Powdered Mix Low Calorie With Aspartame ☛ Serving size= 1 tsp, 8 g; GI= 68 (Medium); GL= 4.7 (Low); Net carb= 7 g

Fruit-Flavored Drink—Powder With High Vitamin C With Other Added Vitamins Low Calorie ☛ Serving size= 1 tsp, 2 g; GI= 68 (Medium); GL= 1.2 (Low); Net carb= 1.8 g

Grape Soda ☛ Serving size= 1 fl oz, 31 g; GI= 68 (Medium); GL= 2.4 (Low); Net carb= 3.5 g

Green Tea ☛ Serving size= 16 fl oz, 473 g; GI= 0 (Low); GL= 0 (Low); Net carb= 0 g

Horchata ☛ Serving size= 1 cup, 228 g; GI= 31 (Low); GL= 8.1 (Low); Net carb= 26.3 g

Ice Mocha ☛ Serving size= 1 cup, 265 g; GI= 21 (Low); GL= 6.4 (Low); Net carb= 30.3 g

Iced Coffee—Brewed ☛ Serving size= 1 fl oz, 30 g; GI= 0 (Low); GL= 0 (Low); Net carb= 0 g

Iced Coffee—Brewed—Decaffeinated ☛ Serving size= 1 fl oz, 30 g; GI= 0 (Low); GL= 0 (Low); Net carb= 0 g

Iced Coffee—Cafe Mocha ☛ Serving size= 1 fl oz, 31 g; GI= 21 (Low); GL= 0.6 (Low); Net carb= 2.8 g

Iced Coffee—Cafe Mocha Decaffeinated ☛ Serving size= 1 fl oz, 31 g; GI= 21 (Low); GL= 0.6 (Low); Net carb= 2.8 g

Iced Coffee—Cafe Mocha Decaffeinated Nonfat ☛ Serving size= 1 fl oz, 31 g; GI= 21 (Low); GL= 0.6 (Low); Net carb= 2.8 g

Iced Coffee—Latte ☛ Serving size= 1 fl oz, 30 g; GI= 21 (Low); GL= 0.2 (Low); Net carb= 0.8 g

Instant Coffee—(Made With Water) ☛ Serving size= 1 fl oz, 29.8 g; GI= 0 (Low); GL= 0 (Low); Net carb= 0.1 g

Lemonade-Flavor Drink Powder Made With Water ☛ Serving size= 1 fl oz, 31.8 g; GI= 68 (Medium); GL= 1.5 (Low); Net carb= 2.2 g

Lemonade—Frozen—Concentrate—Pink Made With Water ☛ Serving size= 1 fl oz, 30.9 g; GI= 68 (Medium); GL= 2.3 (Low); Net carb= 3.3 g

Lemonade—Frozen—Concentrate—White Made With Water ☛ Serving size= 1 fl oz, 30.9 g; GI= 68 (Medium); GL= 2.2 (Low); Net carb= 3.2 g

Lemonade—Fruit Flavored Drink ☛ Serving size= 1 fl oz (no ice), 31 g; GI= 68 (Medium); GL= 1.4 (Low); Net carb= 2 g

Lemonade—Fruit Juice Drink—Light Enriched With Vitamin E And C ☛ Serving size= 8 fl oz, 240 g; GI= 68 (Medium); GL= 8.2 (Low); Net carb= 12 g

Lemonade—Powder Made With Water ☛ Serving size= 1 fl oz, 33 g; GI= 68 (Medium); GL= 0.8 (Low); Net carb= 1.2 g

Limeade Frozen—Concentrate—Made With Water ☛ Serving size= 1 fl oz, 30.9 g; GI= 68 (Medium); GL= 2.9 (Low); Net carb= 4.3 g

Low Calorie Cola ☛ Serving size= 1 fl oz, 29.6 g; GI= 0 (Low); GL= 0 (Low); Net carb= 0 g

Malt Liquor Beverage ☛ Serving size= 1 bottle, 1184 g; GI= 0 (Low); GL= 0 (Low); Net carb= 0 g

Mixed Berry Powerade Zero ☛ Serving size= 12 fl oz, 360 g; GI= 0 (Low); GL= 0 (Low); Net carb= 0.5 g

Oatmeal Beverage—With Water ☛ Serving size= 1 fl oz, 31 g; GI= 59 (Medium); GL= 1.9 (Low); Net carb= 3.2 g

Orange Breakfast Drink—Ready-To-Drink—With Added Nutrients ☛ Serving size= 1 fl oz, 31.6 g; GI= 68 (Medium); GL= 2.8 (Low); Net carb= 4.1 g

Orange Drink—Breakfast Type With Juice And Pulp Frozen Concentrate ☛ Serving size= 1 fl oz, 36.3 g; GI= 68 (Medium); GL= 9.6 (Low); Net carb= 14.1 g

Orange Drink—Breakfast Type With Juice And Pulp Frozen—Concentrate—Made With Water ☛ Serving size= 1 fl oz, 31.3 g; GI= 68 (Medium); GL= 2.4 (Low); Net carb= 3.5 g

Orange Drink—Canned With Added Vitamin C ☛ Serving size= 1 fl oz, 31 g; GI= 68 (Medium); GL= 2.6 (Low); Net carb= 3.8 g

Orange Soda ☛ Serving size= 1 fl oz, 31 g; GI= 68 (Medium); GL= 2.6 (Low); Net carb= 3.8 g

Orange-Flavor Drink—Breakfast Type Low Calorie Powder ☛

Serving size= 1 portion, amount of dry mix to make 8 fl oz Made, 2.5 g; GI= 89 (High); GL= 1.8 (Low); Net carb= 2.1 g

Orange-Flavor Drink—Breakfast Type Powder Made With Water ☛ Serving size= 1 fl oz, 33.9 g; GI= 68 (Medium); GL= 2.9 (Low); Net carb= 4.3 g

Orange-Flavor Drink—Breakfast Type With Pulp Frozen—Concentrate—Made With Water ☛ Serving size= 1 fl oz, 31 g; GI= 68 (Medium); GL= 2.6 (Low); Net carb= 3.8 g

Pepper Soda ☛ Serving size= 1 fl oz, 30.7 g; GI= 68 (Medium); GL= 2.2 (Low); Net carb= 3.2 g

Rich Chocolate Powder ☛ Serving size= 2 tbsp, 11 g; GI= 89 (High); GL= 9.1 (Low); Net carb= 10.2 g

Soy Protein Powder ☛ Serving size= 1 scoop, 44 g; GI= 47 (Low); GL= 9.1 (Low); Net carb= 19.3 g

Sweetened Vanilla Almond Milk ☛ Serving size= 8 fl oz, 240 g; GI= 33 (Low); GL= 4.9 (Low); Net carb= 14.9 g

Tap Water ☛ Serving size= 1 fl oz, 29.6 g; GI= 0 (Low); GL= 0 (Low); Net carb= 0 g

Tea Green Instant Decaffeinated Lemon Unsweetened Enriched With Vitamin C ☛ Serving size= 2 tbsp, 4.5 g; GI= 89 (High); GL= 3.8 (Low); Net carb= 4.3 g

Tea Green—Brewed—Decaffeinated ☛ Serving size= ml, 240 g; GI= 0 (Low); GL= 0 (Low); Net carb= 0 g

Tea Green—Brewed—Regular ☛ Serving size= 1 cup, 245 g; GI= 0 (Low); GL= 0 (Low); Net carb= 0 g

Tea—Black (Brewed) ☛ Serving size= 1 fl oz, 29.6 g; GI= 0 (Low); GL= 0 (Low); Net carb= 0.1 g

Tea—Black (Ready To Drink) ☛ Serving size= 16 fl oz, 473 g; GI= 0 (Low); GL= 0 (Low); Net carb= 0 g

Tea—Black Ready To Drink Decaffeinated Diet ☛ Serving size= 1 cup, 240 g; GI= 0 (Low); GL= 0 (Low); Net carb= 2 g

Tea—Black—Brewed—Made With Distilled Water ☛ Serving size= 1 fl oz, 29.6 g; GI= 0 (Low); GL= 0 (Low); Net carb= 0.1 g

Tea—Black—Brewed—Made With Tap Water Decaffeinated ☛ Serving size= 1 fl oz, 29.6 g; GI= 0 (Low); GL= 0 (Low); Net carb= 0.1 g

Tea—Black—Ready-To-Drink—Lemon (Lipton Brisk) ☛ Serving size= 1 fl oz, 30.6 g; GI= 68 (Medium); GL= 1.8 (Low); Net carb= 2.7 g

Tea—Black—Ready-To-Drink—Lemon Diet ☛ Serving size= 1 cup, 265 g; GI= 0 (Low); GL= 0 (Low); Net carb= 0.6 g

Tea—Black—Ready-To-Drink—Peach Diet ☛ Serving size= 1 cup, 268 g; GI= 0 (Low); GL= 0 (Low); Net carb= 0.7 g

Tea—Herb Other Than Chamomile Brewed ☛ Serving size= 1 fl oz, 29.6 g; GI= 0 (Low); GL= 0 (Low); Net carb= 0.1 g

Tea—Herb—Brewed—Chamomile ☛ Serving size= 1 fl oz, 29.6 g; GI= 0 (Low); GL= 0 (Low); Net carb= 0.1 g

Tea—Hibiscus Brewed ☛ Serving size= 8 fl oz, 237 g; GI= 0 (Low); GL= 0 (Low); Net carb= 0 g

Tea—Hot Chai With Milk ☛ Serving size= 1 fl oz, 30 g; GI= 41 (Low); GL= 1.1 (Low); Net carb= 2.7 g

Water Non-Carbonated Bottles Natural Fruit Flavors Sweetened With Low Calorie Sweetener ☛ Serving size= 1 fl oz, 29.6 g; GI= 0 (Low); GL= 0 (Low); Net carb= 0 g

Whey Protein Powder ☛ Serving size= 2 scoop, 39 g; GI= 47 (Low); GL= 3.3 (Low); Net carb= 7 g

Wine Non-Alcoholic ☛ Serving size= 1 fl oz, 29 g; GI= 7 (Low); GL= 0 (Low); Net carb= 0.3 g

29

CONDIMENTS, OILS & SAUCES

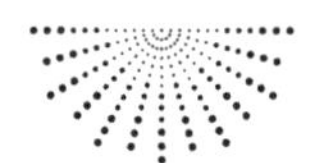

Sauce—Alfredo ☛ Serving size= ¼ cup, 62 g; GI= 27 (Low); GL= 0.4 (Low); Net carb= 1.6 g

Beef Tallow ☛ Serving size= 1 tbsp, 15 g; GI= 0 (Low); GL= 0 (Low); Net carb= 0 g

Clarified Butter ☛ Serving size= 1 tbsp, 15 g; GI= 0 (Low); GL= 0 (Low); Net carb= 0 g

Cocktail sauce ☛ Serving size= ¼ cup, 62 g; GI= 38 (Low); GL= 6.8 (Low); Net carb= 18 g

Dressing—Blue or roquefort ☛ Serving size= 2 tbsp, 30 g; GI= 50 (Low); GL= 4.1 (Low); Net carb= 8.1 g

Dressing—Blue or roquefort, low-calorie ☛ Serving size= 2 tbsp, 30 g; GI= 5 (Low); GL= 0 (Low); Net carb= 0.9 g

Dressing—Blue or roquefort, reduced calorie ☛ Serving size= 2 tbsp, 30 g; GI= 5 (Low); GL= 0 (Low); Net carb= 0.9 g

Dressing—Blue or roquefort, reduced calorie, fat-free ☛ Serving size= 2 tbsp, 30 g; GI= 5 (Low); GL= 0 (Low); Net carb= 0.9 g

Dressing—Caesar ☛ Serving size= ¼ cup, 62 g; GI= 50 (Low); GL= 0.8 (Low); Net carb= 1.6 g

Dressing—Caesar, low-calorie ☛ Serving size= ¼ cup, 62 g; GI= 5 (Low); GL= 0 (Low); Net carb= 0.2 g

Dressing—Coleslaw ☛ Serving size= ¼ cup, 62 g; GI= 50 (Low); GL= 1.2 (Low); Net carb= 2.3 g

Dressing—Coleslaw, reduced calorie ☛ Serving size= ¼ cup, 62 g; GI= 5 (Low); GL= 0 (Low); Net carb= 0 g

Dressing—Cream cheese ☛ Serving size= 2 tbsp, 30 g; GI= 50 (Low); GL= 0.5 (Low); Net carb= 1 g

Dressing—Feta Cheese ☛ Serving size= ¼ cup, 62 g; GI= 50 (Low); GL= 0.7 (Low); Net carb= 1.4 g

Dressing—French ☛ Serving size= 2 tbsp, 30 g; GI= 50 (Low); GL= 4.5 (Low); Net carb= 9 g

Dressing—French, reduced calorie ☛ Serving size= 2 tbsp, 30 g; GI= 50 (Low); GL= 1.9 (Low); Net carb= 3.8 g

Dressing—French, reduced calorie, fat free ☛ Serving size= 2 tbsp, 30 g; GI= 50 (Low); GL= 1.9 (Low); Net carb= 3.8 g

Dressing—Green Goddess ☛ Serving size= 2 tbsp, 30 g; GI= 50 (Low); GL= 1.2 (Low); Net carb= 2.4 g

Dressing—Honey mustard ☛ Serving size= 2 tbsp, 30 g; GI= 50 (Low); GL= 4.2 (Low); Net carb= 8.4 g

Dressing—Honey mustard ☛ Serving size= ¼ cup, 62 g; GI= (Low); GL= 0 (Low); Net carb= 16.8 g

Dressing—Italian dressing ☛ Serving size= 2 tbsp, 30 g; GI= 50 (Low); GL= 1.1 (Low); Net carb= 2.2 g

Dressing—Italian, diet or reduced calorie ☛ Serving size= 2 tbsp, 30 g; GI= 5 (Low); GL= 0 (Low); Net carb= 0.4 g

Dressing—Italian, diet or reduced calorie, fat free ☛ Serving size= 2 tbsp, 30 g; GI= 5 (Low); GL= 0 (Low); Net carb= 0.4 g

Dressing—Italian, reduced calorie ☛ Serving size= 2 tbsp, 30 g; GI= 5 (Low); GL= 0 (Low); Net carb= 0.4 g

Dressing—Korean ☛ Serving size= ¼ cup, 62 g; GI= 50 (Low); GL= 1.9 (Low); Net carb= 3.7 g

Dressing—Mayonnaise-type salad, cholesterol-free ☛ Serving size= 2 tbsp, 30 g; GI= 50 (Low); GL= 3 (Low); Net carb= 6 g

Dressing—Mayonnaise-type salad, diet ☛ Serving size= 2 tbsp, 30 g; GI= 50 (Low); GL= 1.1 (Low); Net carb= 2.2 g

Dressing—Milk, vinegar based ☛ Serving size= 2 tbsp, 30 g; GI= 50 (Low); GL= 1 (Low); Net carb= 1.9 g

Dressing—Peppercorn ☛ Serving size= 2 tbsp, 30 g; GI= 50 (Low); GL= 1 (Low); Net carb= 2 g

Dressing—Peppercorn ☛ Serving size= ¼ cup, 62 g; GI= 50 (Low); GL= 2 (Low); Net carb= 4 g

Dressing—Poppy seed ☛ Serving size= ¼ cup, 62 g; GI= 50 (Low); GL= 6.2 (Low); Net carb= 12.4 g

Dressing—Poppy seed ☛ Serving size= 2 tbsp, 30 g; GI= 50 (Low); GL= 3.1 (Low); Net carb= 6.2 g

Dressing—Rice ☛ Serving size= ¼ cup, 62 g; GI= 64 (Low); GL= 6.7 (Low); Net carb= 10.5 g

Dressing—Rice ☛ Serving size= 2 tbsp, 30 g; GI= 64 (Low); GL= 3.4 (Low); Net carb= 5.3 g

Dressing—Russian ☛ Serving size= ¼ cup, 62 g; GI= 50 (Low); GL= 9.7 (Low); Net carb= 19.3 g

Dressing—Russian ☛ Serving size= 2 tbsp, 30 g; GI= 50 (Low); GL= 4.8 (Low); Net carb= 9.6 g

Dressing—Salad, common ☛ Serving size= ¼ cup, 62 g; GI= 50 (Low); GL= 2.8 (Low); Net carb= 5.6 g

Dressing—Salad, common ☛ Serving size= 2 tbsp, 30 g; GI= 50 (Low); GL= 1.4 (Low); Net carb= 2.8 g

Dressing—Sesame ☛ Serving size= ¼ cup, 62 g; GI= 50 (Low); GL= 7.4 (Low); Net carb= 14.8 g

Dressing—Sesame ☛ Serving size= 2 tbsp, 30 g; GI= 50 (Low); GL= 3.7 (Low); Net carb= 7.4 g

Dressing—Sweet and sour ☛ Serving size= ¼ cup, 62 g; GI= 50 (Low); GL= 1.2 (Low); Net carb= 2.4 g

Dressing—Thousand Island Regular ☛ Serving size= 2 tbsp, 30 g; GI= 50 (Low); GL= 1.5 (Low); Net carb= 2.9 g

Dressing—Thousand Island Regular ☛ Serving size= ¼ cup, 62 g; GI= 50 (Low); GL= 2.9 (Low); Net carb= 5.8 g

Dressing—Vinegar based ☛ Serving size= ¼ cup, 62 g; GI= 50 (Low); GL= 0.8 (Low); Net carb= 1.6 g

Dressing—Yogurt ☛ Serving size= ¼ cup, 62 g; GI= 50 (Low); GL= 1.9 (Low); Net carb= 3.8 g

Dressing—Yogurt ☛ Serving size= 2 tbsp, 30 g; GI= 50 (Low); GL= 1 (Low); Net carb= 1.9 g

Duck Fat ☛ Serving size= 2 tbsp, 30 g; GI= 0 (Low); GL= 0 (Low); Net carb= 0 g

Mayonnaise (mean value) ☛ Serving size= 2 tbsp, 30 g; GI= 50 (Low); GL= 1.2 (Low); Net carb= 2.4 g

Mayonnaise—made with tofu ☛ Serving size= 2 tbsp, 30 g; GI= 50 (Low); GL= 0.3 (Low); Net carb= 0.6 g

Mustard greens (mean value) ☛ Serving size= 2 tbsp, 30 g; GI= 32 (Low); GL= 0.2 (Low); Net carb= 0.5 g

Mustard pickles ☛ Serving size= 2 tbsp, 30 g; GI= 32 (Low); GL= 2.4 (Low); Net carb= 7.5 g

Oil—Avocado ☛ Serving size= 2 tbsp, 30 g; GI= 0 (Low); GL= 0 (Low); Net carb= 0 g

Oil—Canola ☛ Serving size= 2 tbsp, 30 g; GI= 0 (Low); GL= 0 (Low); Net carb= 0 g

Oil—Coconut ☛ Serving size= 2 tbsp, 30 g; GI= 0 (Low); GL= 0 (Low); Net carb= 0 g

Oil—Corn ☛ Serving size= 2 tbsp, 30 g; GI= 0 (Low); GL= 0 (Low); Net carb= 0 g

Oil—Extra-virgin olive ☛ Serving size= 2 tbsp, 30 g; GI= 0 (Low); GL= 0 (Low); Net carb= 0 g

Oil—Flaxseed ☛ Serving size= 2 tbsp, 30 g; GI= 0 (Low); GL= 0 (Low); Net carb= 0 g

Oil—Grapeseed ☛ Serving size= 2 tbsp, 30 g; GI= 0 (Low); GL= 0 (Low); Net carb= 0 g

Oil—Hazelnut ☛ Serving size= 2 tbsp, 30 g; GI= 0 (Low); GL= 0 (Low); Net carb= 0 g

Oil—Hemp seed ☛ Serving size= 2 tbsp, 30 g; GI= 0 (Low); GL= 0 (Low); Net carb= 0 g

Oil—Macadamia Nut ☛ Serving size= 2 tbsp, 30 g; GI= 0 (Low); GL= 0 (Low); Net carb= 0 g

Oil—Olive ☛ Serving size= 2 tbsp, 30 g; GI= 0 (Low); GL= 0 (Low); Net carb= 0 g

Oil—Palm ☛ Serving size= 2 tbsp, 30 g; GI= 0 (Low); GL= 0 (Low); Net carb= 0 g

Oil—Peanut ☛ Serving size= 2 tbsp, 30 g; GI= 0 (Low); GL= 0 (Low); Net carb= 0 g

Oil—Rice Bran ☛ Serving size= 2 tbsp, 30 g; GI= 0 (Low); GL= 0 (Low); Net carb= 0 g

Oil—Sesame ☛ Serving size= 2 tbsp, 30 g; GI= 0 (Low); GL= 0 (Low); Net carb= 0 g

Oil—Sunflower ☛ Serving size= 2 tbsp, 30 g; GI= 0 (Low); GL= 0 (Low); Net carb= 0 g

Oil—Vegetable ☛ Serving size= 2 tbsp, 30 g; GI= 0 (Low); GL= 0 (Low); Net carb= 0 g

Oil—Walnut ☛ Serving size= 2 tbsp, 30 g; GI= 0 (Low); GL= 0 (Low); Net carb= 0 g

Vinegar, sugar, and water dressing ☛ Serving size= 2 tbsp, 30 g; GI= 0 (Low); GL= 0 (Low); Net carb= 0 g

30
DAIRY AND SOY ALTERNATIVES

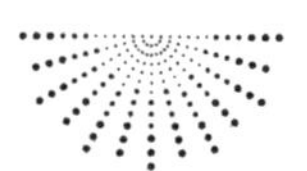

Butter-margarine blend, stick, salted ☛ Serving size: 1 tsp (4.7 g); GI= 50 (Low); GL= 0.3 (Low); Net carb= 0.6 g

Butter-margarine blend, stick, unsalted ☛ Serving size: 1 tsp (4.7 g); GI= 50 (Low); GL= 0.3 (Low); Net carb= 0.6 g

Butter-vegetable oil blend ☛ Serving size: 1 tsp (4.7 g); GI= 50 (Low); GL= 0.3 (Low); Net carb= 0.6 g

Butter—Light, whipped, tub, salted ☛ Serving size: 1 tsp (4.7 g); GI= 0 (Low); GL= 0 (Low); Net carb= 0 g

Butter, minimally processed ☛ Serving size: 1 tsp (4.7 g); GI= 50 (Low); GL= 0.3 (Low); Net carb= 0.6 g

Butter, stick, salted ☛ Serving size: 1 tsp (4.7 g); GI= 50 (Low); GL= 0.3 (Low); Net carb= 0.6 g

Butter, stick, unsalted ☛ Serving size: 1 tsp (4.7 g); GI= 50 (Low); GL= 0.3 (Low); Net carb= 0.6 g

Buttermilk, fluid, 2% fat ☛ Serving size: 1 cup (245 g); GI= 29.5 (Low); GL= 3.6 (Low); Net carb= 12.2 g

Buttermilk, fluid, nonfat ☛ Serving size: 1 cup (245 g); GI= 32 (Low); GL= 3.9 (Low); Net carb= 12.2 g

Carry-out milk shake, chocolate ☛ Serving size: 1 cup (245 g); GI= 44 (Low); GL= 5.4 (Low); Net carb= 12.3 g

Carry-out milk shake, flavors other than chocolate ☛ Serving size: 1 cup (245 g); GI= 44 (Low); GL= 5.4 (Low); Net carb= 12.3 g

Cheese—Amercican style ☛ Serving size: 1 oz (28.35 g); GI= 27 (Low); GL= 0.2 (Low); Net carb= 0.7 g

Cheese—Blue ☛ Serving size: 1 oz (28.35 g); GI= 0.0 (Low); GL= 0 (Low); Net carb= 0 g

Cheese—camembert ☛ Serving size: 1 oz (28.35 g); GI= 25 (Low); GL= 0.2 (Low); Net carb= 0.8 g

Cheese—cheddar ☛ Serving size: 1 oz (28.35 g); GI= 27 (Low); GL= 0.2 (Low); Net carb= 0.7 g

Cheese—Colby ☛ Serving size: 1 oz (28.35 g); GI= 27 (Low); GL= 0.2 (Low); Net carb= 0.7 g

Cheese—cottage, low-fat ☛ Serving size: 1 oz (28.35 g); GI= 10 (Low); GL= 0.1 (Low); Net carb= 1 g

Cheese—cottage, minimally processed ☛ Serving size: 1 oz (28.35 g); GI= 29.5 (Low); GL= 0.3 (Low); Net carb= 1 g

Cheese—cottage, regular-fat ☛ Serving size: 1 oz (28.35 g); GI= 10 (Low); GL= 0.1 (Low); Net carb= 1 g

Cheese—cottage, salted, dry curd ☛ Serving size: 1 oz (28.35 g); GI= 32 (Low); GL= 0.3 (Low); Net carb= 0.9 g

Cheese—cottage, with fruit ☛ Serving size: 1 oz (28.35 g); GI= 42.5 (Low); GL= 0.4 (Low); Net carb= 0.9 g

Cheese—cream ☛ Serving size: 1 oz (28.35 g); GI= 27 (Low); GL= 2.3 (Low); Net carb= 8.5 g

Cheese—cream, lowfat ☛ Serving size: 1 oz (28.35 g); GI= 27 (Low); GL= 2.3 (Low); Net carb= 8.5 g

Cheese—Edam ☛ Serving size: 1 oz (28.35 g); GI= 27 (Low); GL= 0.2 (Low); Net carb= 0.7 g

Cheese—Feta ☛ Serving size: 1 oz (28.35 g); GI= 27 (Low); GL= 0.2 (Low); Net carb= 0.7 g

Cheese—Fontina ☛ Serving size: 1 oz (28.35 g); GI= 27 (Low); GL= 0.2 (Low); Net carb= 0.7 g

Cheese—goat ☛ Serving size: 1 oz (28.35 g); GI= 27 (Low); GL= 0.2 (Low); Net carb= 0.7 g

Cheese—Gouda ☛ Serving size: 1 oz (28.35 g); GI= 27 (Low); GL= 0.2 (Low); Net carb= 0.7 g

Cheese—Gruyere ☛ Serving size: 1 oz (28.35 g); GI= 27 (Low); GL= 0.2 (Low); Net carb= 0.7 g

Cheese—halloumi ☛ Serving size: 1 oz (28.35 g); GI= 0.0 (Low); GL= 0 (Low); Net carb= 0 g

Cheese—havarti ☛ Serving size: 1 oz (28.35 g); GI= 0.0 (Low); GL= 0 (Low); Net carb= 0 g

Cheese—Limburger ☛ Serving size: 1 oz (28.35 g); GI= 27 (Low); GL= 0.2 (Low); Net carb= 0.7 g

Cheese—Manchego ☛ Serving size: 1 oz (28.35 g); GI= 27 (Low); GL= 0.2 (Low); Net carb= 0.7 g

Cheese—Monterey ☛ Serving size: 1 oz (28.35 g); GI= 27 (Low); GL= 0.2 (Low); Net carb= 0.7 g

Cheese—mozzarella ☛ Serving size: 1 oz (28.35 g); GI= 27 (Low); GL= 0.2 (Low); Net carb= 0.7 g

Cheese—Mozzarella, low sodium ☛ Serving size: 1 oz (28.35 g); GI= 27 (Low); GL= 0.2 (Low); Net carb= 0.7 g

Cheese—Mozzarella, average value ☛ Serving size: 1 oz (28.35 g); GI= 27 (Low); GL= 0.2 (Low); Net carb= 0.7 g

Cheese—Mozzarella, nonfat or fat free ☛ Serving size: 1 oz (28.35 g); GI= 32 (Low); GL= 0.3 (Low); Net carb= 0.9 g

Cheese—Mozzarella, part skim ☛ Serving size: 1 oz (28.35 g); GI= 27 (Low); GL= 0.2 (Low); Net carb= 0.7 g

Cheese—Muenster ☛ Serving size: 1 oz (28.35 g); GI= 27 (Low); GL= 0.2 (Low); Net carb= 0.7 g

Cheese—Muenster, lowfat ☛ Serving size: 1 oz (28.35 g); GI= 27 (Low); GL= 0.2 (Low); Net carb= 0.7 g

Cheese—natural, Cheddar or American type ☛ Serving size: 1 oz (28.35 g); GI= 27 (Low); GL= 0.2 (Low); Net carb= 0.7 g

Cheese—natural, minimally processed ☛ Serving size: 1 oz (28.35 g); GI= 27 (Low); GL= 0.2 (Low); Net carb= 0.7 g

Cheese—minimally processed ☛ Serving size: 1 oz (28.35 g); GI= 27 (Low); GL= 0.2 (Low); Net carb= 0.7 g

Cheese—Parmesan ☛ Serving size: 1 oz (28.35 g); GI= 27 (Low); GL= 0.2 (Low); Net carb= 0.7 g

Cheese—Parmesan, dry grated ☛ Serving size: 1 oz (28.35 g); GI= 27 (Low); GL= 0.2 (Low); Net carb= 0.7 g

Cheese—Parmesan, hard ☛ Serving size: 1 oz (28.35 g); GI= 27 (Low); GL= 0.2 (Low); Net carb= 0.7 g

Cheese—Parmesan, low sodium ☛ Serving size: 1 oz (28.35 g); GI= 27 (Low); GL= 0.2 (Low); Net carb= 0.7 g

Cheese—Pecorino Romano ☛ Serving size: 1 oz (28.35 g); GI= 0.0 (Low); GL= 0 (Low); Net carb= 0 g

Cheese—processed cheese common ☛ Serving size: 1 oz (28.35 g); GI= 27 (Low); GL= 1.2 (Low); Net carb= 4.4 g

Cheese—processed cheese, American type based ☛ Serving size: 1 oz (28.35 g); GI= 27 (Low); GL= 1.2 (Low); Net carb= 4.4 g

Cheese—processed cheese, Cheddar based ☛ Serving size: 1 oz (28.35 g); GI= 27 (Low); GL= 1.2 (Low); Net carb= 4.4 g

Cheese—processed cheese, Swiss based ☛ Serving size: 1 oz (28.35 g); GI= 27 (Low); GL= 1.2 (Low); Net carb= 4.4 g

Cheese—processed cream cheese ☛ Serving size: 1 oz (28.35 g); GI= 32 (Low); GL= 1.5 (Low); Net carb= 4.7 g

Cheese—processed, American and Swiss cheese based ☛ Serving size: 1 oz (28.35 g); GI= 27 (Low); GL= 1.2 (Low); Net carb= 4.4 g

Cheese—processed, American or Cheddar type based low fat ☛ Serving size: 1 oz (28.35 g); GI= 27 (Low); GL= 1.2 (Low); Net carb= 4.4 g

Cheese—processed, American or Cheddar type based, fat free ☛ Serving size: 1 oz (28.35 g); GI= 32 (Low); GL= 1.5 (Low); Net carb= 4.7 g

Cheese—processed, American or Cheddar type based, low sodium ☛ Serving size: 1 oz (28.35 g); GI= 27 (Low); GL= 1.2 (Low); Net carb= 4.4 g

Cheese—processed, made with vegetables ☛ Serving size: 1 oz (28.35 g); GI= 27 (Low); GL= 1.2 (Low); Net carb= 4.4 g

Cheese—processed, Mozzarella based, low sodium ☛ Serving size: 1 oz (28.35 g); GI= 27 (Low); GL= 1.2 (Low); Net carb= 4.4 g

Cheese—processed, Swiss cheese based ☛ Serving size: 1 oz (28.35 g); GI= 27 (Low); GL= 1.2 (Low); Net carb= 4.4 g

Cheese—processed, Swiss cheese based, low sodium ☛ Serving size: 1 oz (28.35 g); GI= 27 (Low); GL= 1.2 (Low); Net carb= 4.4 g

Cheese—processed, Swiss cheese based, lowfat ☛ Serving size: 1 oz (28.35 g); GI= 27 (Low); GL= 1.2 (Low); Net carb= 4.4 g

Cheese—processed, Swiss cheese based, lowfat, low sodium ☛ Serving size: 1 oz (28.35 g); GI= 27 (Low); GL= 1.2 (Low); Net carb= 4.4 g

Cheese—processed,Colby, , based low fat, low sodium ☛ Serving size: 1 oz (28.35 g); GI= 27 (Low); GL= 1.2 (Low); Net carb= 4.4 g

Cheese—Provolone ☛ Serving size: 1 oz (28.35 g); GI= 27 (Low); GL= 0.2 (Low); Net carb= 0.7 g

Cheese—Ricotta ☛ Serving size: 1 oz (28.35 g); GI= 27 (Low); GL= 0.2 (Low); Net carb= 0.7 g

Cheese—Roquefort ☛ Serving size: 1 oz (28.35 g); GI= 0.0 (Low); GL= 0 (Low); Net carb= 0 g

Cheese—Semi-soft, low sodium ☛ Serving size: 1 oz (28.35 g); GI= 27 (Low); GL= 0.2 (Low); Net carb= 0.7 g

Cheese—Swiss ☛ Serving size: 1 oz (28.35 g); GI= 27 (Low); GL= 0.2 (Low); Net carb= 0.7 g

Cheese—Swiss, low sodium ☛ Serving size: 1 oz (28.35 g); GI= 27 (Low); GL= 0.2 (Low); Net carb= 0.7 g

Cheese—Swiss, lowfat ☛ Serving size: 1 oz (28.35 g); GI= 27 (Low); GL= 0.2 (Low); Net carb= 0.7 g

Cow's—Milk skim ☛ Serving size: 1 cup (245 g); GI= 40 (Low); GL= 4.8 (Low); Net carb= 12 g

Cow's—Milk full cream ☛ Serving size: 1 cup (245 g); GI= 40 (Low); GL= 4.8 (Low); Net carb= 12 g

Cream cheese ☛ Serving size: 1 oz (28.35 g); GI= 0.0 (Low); GL= 0 (Low); Net carb= 0 g

Cream substitute—frozen ☛ Serving size: 1 oz (28.35 g); GI= 27 (Low); GL= 2.3 (Low); Net carb= 8.5 g

Cream substitute—frozen, liquid, and/or powdered ☛ Serving size: 1 oz (28.35g); GI= 27 (Low); GL= 2.3 (Low); Net carb= 8.5 g

Cream substitute—light, liquid ☛ Serving size: 1 oz (28.35 g); GI= 27 (Low); GL= 2.3 (Low); Net carb= 8.5 g

Cream substitute—light, powdered ☛ Serving size: 1 oz (28.35 g); GI= 27 (Low); GL= 2.3 (Low); Net carb= 8.5 g

Cream substitute—liquid ☛ Serving size: 1 oz (28.35 g); GI= 27 (Low); GL= 2.3 (Low); Net carb= 8.5 g

Cream substitute—powdered ☛ Serving size: 1 oz (28.35 g); GI= 27 (Low); GL= 2.3 (Low); Net carb= 8.5 g

Cream—average value, half and half ☛ Serving size: 1 oz (28.35 g); GI= 27 (Low); GL= 2.3 (Low); Net carb= 8.5 g

Cream—half and half ☛ Serving size: 1 oz (28.35 g); GI= 27 (Low); GL= 2.3 (Low); Net carb= 8.5 g

Cream—heavy, fluid ☛ Serving size: 1 oz (28.35 g); GI= 27 (Low); GL= 2.3 (Low); Net carb= 8.5 g

Cream—light, fluid ☛ Serving size: 1 oz (28.35 g); GI= 27 (Low); GL= 2.3 (Low); Net carb= 8.5 g

Cream—light, whipped, and unsweetened ☛ Serving size: 1 oz (28.35 g); GI= 27 (Low); GL= 2.3 (Low); Net carb= 8.5 g

Cream—pure regular-fat ☛ Serving size: 1 oz (28.35 g); GI= 0.0 (Low); GL= 0 (Low); Net carb= 0 g

Cream—sour ☛ Serving size: 1 oz (28.35 g); GI= 0.0 (Low); GL= 0 (Low); Net carb= 0 g

Cream—thickened regular-fat ☛ Serving size: 1 oz (28.35 g); GI= 0.0 (Low); GL= 0 (Low); Net carb= 0 g

Cream—whipped ☛ Serving size: 1 oz (28.35 g); GI= 0.0 (Low); GL= 0 (Low); Net carb= 0 g

Custard homemade ☛ Serving size: ½ cup (116 g); GI= 29 (Low); GL= 6.7 (Low); Net carb= 23.1 g

Custard industrially made ☛ Serving size: ½ cup (116 g); GI= 38 (Low); GL= 8.8 (Low); Net carb= 23.2 g

Custard—Puerto Rican style ☛ Serving size: ½ cup (116 g); GI= 38 (Low); GL= 8.8 (Low); Net carb= 23.2 g

Dip—cream cheese base ☛ Serving size: 1 oz (28.35 g); GI= 27 (Low); GL= 9.4 (Low); Net carb= 34.8 g

Dip—sour cream base ☛ Serving size: 1 oz (28.35 g); GI= 27 (Low); GL= 9.4 (Low); Net carb= 34.8 g

Dip—sour cream base, low calorie ☛ Serving size: 1 oz (28.35 g); GI= 27 (Low); GL= 9.4 (Low); Net carb= 34.8 g

Dip, cheese—chili con queso ☛ Serving size: 1 oz (28.35 g); GI= 27 (Low); GL= 9.4 (Low); Net carb= 34.8 g

Ghee ☛ Serving size: 1 tsp (4.7 g); GI= 0.0 (Low); GL= 0 (Low); Net carb= 0 g

Goat—Cheese ☛ Serving size: 1 oz (28.35 g); GI= 27 (Low); GL= 0.2 (Low); Net carb= 0.7 g

Goat—Cheese plain ☛ Serving size: 1 oz (28.35 g); GI= 0.0 (Low); GL= 0 (Low); Net carb= 0 g

Goat's—Milk whole ☛ Serving size: 1 cup (245 g); GI= 40 (Low); GL= 4.4 (Low); Net carb= 11 g

Goat's—milk yoghurt ☛ Serving size: 8 oz (225 g); GI= 25 (Low); GL= 2.75 (Low); Net carb= 11 g

Ice cream—average value ☛ Serving size: 1 scoop (72 g)

; GI= 61 (Medium); GL= 7.5 (Low); Net carb= 12.3 g

Ice cream—bar or stick, not covered by chocolate ☛ Serving size: 1 scoop (72 g)

; GI= 61 (Medium); GL= 7.5 (Low); Net carb= 12.3 g

Ice cream—regular, chocolate ☛ Serving size: 1 scoop (72 g)

; GI= 61 (Medium); GL= 7.5 (Low); Net carb= 12.3 g

Ice cream—regular, flavors other than chocolate ☛ Serving size: 1 scoop (72 g)

; GI= 61 (Medium); GL= 7.5 (Low); Net carb= 12.3 g

Ice cream—rich, chocolate ☛ Serving size: 1 scoop (72 g)

; GI= 37 (Low); GL= 4.5 (Low); Net carb= 12.2 g

Ice cream—rich, flavors other than chocolate ☛ Serving size: 1 scoop (72 g)

; GI= 38 (Low); GL= 4.7 (Low); Net carb= 12.4 g

Ice cream—soda, chocolate ☛ Serving size: 1 scoop (72 g)

; GI= 59.5 (Medium); GL= 7.3 (Low); Net carb= 12.3 g

Ice cream—soda, flavors other than chocolate ☛ Serving size: 1 scoop (72 g)

; GI= 64.5 (Medium); GL= 7.9 (Low); Net carb= 12.2 g

Ice cream—soft serve, average value ☛ Serving size: 1 scoop (72 g)

; GI= 61 (Medium); GL= 7.5 (Low); Net carb= 12.3 g

Ice cream—soft serve, chocolate ☛ Serving size: 1 scoop (72 g)

; GI= 61 (Medium); GL= 7.5 (Low); Net carb= 12.3 g

Ice cream—soft serve, flavors other than chocolate ☛ Serving size: 1 scoop (72 g)

; GI= 61 (Medium); GL= 7.5 (Low); Net carb= 12.3 g

Ice cream—with sherbet ☛ Serving size: 1 scoop (72 g)

; GI= 51.5 (Low); GL= 6.3 (Low); Net carb= 12.2 g

Ice-cream ☛ Serving size: 1 scoop (72 g)

; GI= 63 (; GL= 7.7 (Low); Net carb= 12.2 g

Imitation cheese—American type ☛ Serving size: 1 oz (28.35 g); GI= 27 (Low); GL= 1.8 (Low); Net carb= 6.7 g

Imitation cheese—cheddar ☛ Serving size: 1 oz (28.35 g); GI= 27 (Low); GL= 1.8 (Low); Net carb= 6.7 g

Imitation cheese—Edam ☛ Serving size: 1 oz (28.35 g); GI= 27 (Low); GL= 1.8 (Low); Net carb= 6.7 g

Imitation cheese—Mozzarella ☛ Serving size: 1 oz (28.35 g); GI= 27 (Low); GL= 1.8 (Low); Net carb= 6.7 g

Kefir ☛ Serving size: 1 cup (245 g); GI= 32 (Low); GL= 0.7 (Low); Net carb= 2.2 g

Light ice cream—chocolate ☛ Serving size: 1 scoop (72 g)

; GI= 50 (Low); GL= 3.4 (Low); Net carb= 6.8 g

Light ice cream—flavors other than chocolate ☛ Serving size: 1 scoop (72 g)

; GI= 50 (Low); GL= 3.4 (Low); Net carb= 6.8 g

Light ice cream—fudgesicle ☛ Serving size: 1 scoop (72 g)

; GI= 50 (Low); GL= 3.4 (Low); Net carb= 6.8 g

Light ice cream—NFS ☛ Serving size: 1 scoop (72 g)

; GI= 50 (Low); GL= 3.4 (Low); Net carb= 6.8 g

Light ice cream—premium, chocolate ☛ Serving size: 1 scoop (72 g)

; GI= 50 (Low); GL= 3.4 (Low); Net carb= 6.8 g

Light ice cream—premium, flavors other than chocolate ☛ Serving size: 1 scoop (72 g); GI= 50 (Low); GL= 3.4 (Low); Net carb= 6.8 g

Light ice cream—soft serve, chocolate ☛ Serving size: 1 scoop (72 g); GI= 50 (Low); GL= 3.4 (Low); Net carb= 6.8 g

Light ice cream—soft serve, flavors other than chocolate ☛ Serving size: 1 scoop (72 g); GI= 50 (Low); GL= 3.4 (Low); Net carb= 6.8 g

Light ice cream—with sherbet ☛ Serving size: 1 scoop (72 g); GI= 46 (Low); GL= 3.1 (Low); Net carb= 6.7 g

Margarine—common ☛ Serving size: 1 tsp (4.7 g); GI= 0 (Low); GL= 0 (Low); Net carb= 0 g

Margarine—stick, salted ☛ Serving size: 1 tsp (4.7 g); GI= 50 (Low); GL= 0 (Low); Net carb= 0 g

Margarine—stick, unsalted ☛ Serving size: 1 tsp (4.7 g); GI= 50 (Low); GL= 0 (Low); Net carb= 0 g

Margarine—tub, salted ☛ Serving size: 1 tsp (4.7 g); GI= 50 (Low); GL= 0 (Low); Net carb= 0 g

Margarine—tub, unsalted ☛ Serving size: 1 tsp (4.7 g); GI= 50 (Low); GL= 0 (Low); Net carb= 0 g

Margarine—whipped, stick, salted ☛ Serving size: 1 tsp (4.7 g); GI= 50 (Low); GL= 0 (Low); Net carb= 0 g

Margarine—whipped, tub, salted ☛ Serving size: 1 tsp (4.7 g); GI= 50 (Low); GL= 0 (Low); Net carb= 0 g

Margarine—whipped, tub, unsalted ☛ Serving size: 1 tsp (4.7 g); GI= 50 (Low); GL= 0 (Low); Net carb= 0 g

Milk beverage—nonfat dry milk, chocolate and low calorie sweetener ☛ Serving size: 1 cup (245 g); GI= 24 (Low); GL= 2.6 (Low); Net carb= 10.8 g

Milk beverage—whole milk, flavors other than chocolate ☛ Serving size: 1 cup (245 g); GI= 35 (Low); GL= 3.9 (Low); Net carb= 11.1 g

Milk dessert—frozen, chocolate (no butterfat) ☛ Serving size: ½ cup (68 g); GI= 61 (Medium); GL= 6.6 (Low); Net carb= 10.8 g

Milk dessert—frozen, flavors other than chocolate ☛ Serving size: ½ cup (68 g); GI= 61 (Medium); GL= 6.6 (Low); Net carb= 10.8 g

Milk dessert—frozen, low-calorie sweetener ☛ Serving size: ½ cup (68 g); GI= 50 (Low); GL= 5.4 (Low); Net carb= 10.8 g

Milk lactose—free ☛ Serving size: 1 cup (245 g); GI= 40 (Low); GL= 6 (Low); Net carb= 15 g

Milk made from soy protein ☛ Serving size: 1 cup (245 g); GI= 50 (Low); GL= 7.4 (Low); Net carb= 14.8 g

Milk—chocolate, average value ☛ Serving size: 1 cup (245 g); GI= 37 (Low); GL= 9.1 (Low); Net carb= 24.6 g

Milk—chocolate, skim ☛ Serving size: 1 cup (245 g); GI= 37.5 (Low); GL= 9.2 (Low); Net carb= 24.5 g

Milk—chocolate, whole ☛ Serving size: 1 cup (245 g); GI= 36 (Low); GL= 8.8 (Low); Net carb= 24.4 g

Milk—cow's, calcium fortified, fluid, 1% fat ☛ Serving size: 1 cup (245 g); GI= 32 (Low); GL= 3.8 (Low); Net carb= 11.9 g

Milk—cow's, calcium fortified, fluid, skim or nonfat ☛ Serving size: 1 cup (245 g); GI= 32 (Low); GL= 3.8 (Low); Net carb= 11.9 g

Milk—cow's, fluid, 1% fat ☛ Serving size: 1 cup (245 g); GI= 32 (Low); GL= 3.8 (Low); Net carb= 11.9 g

Milk—cow's, fluid, 1% fat, acidophilus ☛ Serving size: 1 cup (245 g); GI= 32 (Low); GL= 3.8 (Low); Net carb= 11.9 g

Milk—cow's, fluid, 2% fat ☛ Serving size: 1 cup (245 g); GI= 29.5 (Low); GL= 3.5 (Low); Net carb= 11.9 g

Milk—cow's, fluid, whole ☛ Serving size: 1 cup (245 g); GI= 27 (Low); GL= 3.2 (Low); Net carb= 11.9 g

Milk—dry, reconstituted, 0% fat ☛ Serving size: 1 cup (245 g); GI= 32 (Low); GL= 3.8 (Low); Net carb= 11.9 g

Milk—dry, reconstituted, average value ☛ Serving size: 1 cup (245 g); GI= 32 (Low); GL= 3.8 (Low); Net carb= 11.9 g

Milk—evaporated ☛ Serving size: 1 oz; GI= 40 (Low); GL= 1.2 (Low); Net carb= 3 g

Milk—flavors other than chocolate, whole milk-based ☛ Serving size: 1 cup (245 g); GI= 35 (Low); GL= 4.2 (Low); Net carb= 12 g

Milk—goat's, fluid, whole ☛ Serving size: 1 cup (245 g); GI= 27 (Low); GL= 3.24 (Low); Net carb= 12 g

Milk—imitation, fluid, soy based ☛ Serving size: 1 cup (245 g); GI= 40 (Low); GL= 4.8 (Low); Net carb= 12 g

Milk—malted, fortified, chocolate, made with milk ☛ Serving size: 1 cup (245 g); GI= 45 (Low); GL= 5.4 (Low); Net carb= 12 g

Milk—malted, fortified, natural flavor, made with milk ☛ Serving size: 1 cup (245 g); GI= 45 (Low); GL= 5.4 (Low); Net carb= 12 g

Milk—soy, dry, reconstituted, not baby's ☛ Serving size: 1 cup (245 g); GI= 40 (Low); GL= 5.9 (Low); Net carb= 14.8 g

Milk—soy, ready-to-drink, not baby's ☛ Serving size: 1 cup (245 g); GI= 40 (Low); GL= 5.9 (Low); Net carb= 14.8 g

Milk—vinegar, and sugar dressing ☛ Serving size: 1 cup (245 g); GI= 50 (Low); GL= 7.4 (Low); Net carb= 14.8 g

Milk—whole ☛ Serving size: 1 cup (245 g); GI= 40 (Low); GL= 4.9 (Low); Net carb= 12.3 g

Milk, almond ☛ Serving size: 1 cup (245 g); GI= 25 (Low); GL= 2 (Low); Net carb= 8 g

Milk, coconut ☛ Serving size: 1 cup (245 g); GI= 41 (Low); GL= 6 (Low); Net carb= 14.6 g

Milk, hemp ☛ Serving size: 1 cup (245 g); GI= 0.0 (Low); GL= 0 (Low); Net carb= 0 g

Milk, soy, beans ☛ Serving size: 1 cup (245 g); GI= 41 (Low); GL= 6 (Low); Net carb= 14.6 g

Pudding—canned, chocolate ☛ Serving size: 4 oz (120 g); GI= 44 (Low); GL= 10.6 (Low); Net carb= 24.1 g

Pudding—canned, low calorie, containing artificial sweetener, chocolate ☛ Serving size: 4 oz (120 g); GI= 44 (Low); GL= 10.6 (Low); Net carb= 24.1 g

Pudding—canned, low calorie, containing artificial sweetener, flavors other than chocolate ☛ Serving size: 4 oz (120 g); GI= 44 (Low); GL= 10.6 (Low); Net carb= 24.1 g

Pudding—chocolate, prepared from dry mix, low calorie, containing artificial sweetener, milk added ☛ Serving size: 4 oz (120 g); GI= 44 (Low); GL= 10.6 (Low); Net carb= 24.1 g

Pudding—chocolate, prepared from dry mix, milk added ☛ Serving size: 4 oz (120 g); GI= 44 (Low); GL= 10.6 (Low); Net carb= 24.1 g

Pudding—flavors other than chocolate, prepared from dry mix, low calorie, containing artificial sweetener, milk added ☛ Serving size: 4 oz (120 g); GI= 44 (Low); GL= 10.6 (Low); Net carb= 24.1 g

Pudding—flavors other than chocolate, prepared from dry mix, milk added ☛ Serving size: 4 oz (120 g); GI= 44 (Low); GL= 10.6 (Low); Net carb= 24.1 g

Pudding—pumpkin ☛ Serving size: 4 oz (120 g); GI= 44 (Low); GL= 8.8 (Low); Net carb= 20 g

Quark Cheese ☛ Serving size: 1 oz (28.35 g); GI= 27 (Low); GL= 0.2 (Low); Net carb= 0.7 g

Queso—Anejo (aged cheese) ☛ Serving size: 1 oz (28.35 g); GI= 27 (Low); GL= 0.2 (Low); Net carb= 0.7 g

Queso—Asadero ☛ Serving size: 1 oz (28.35 g); GI= 27 (Low); GL= 0.2 (Low); Net carb= 0.7 g

Queso—Chihuahua ☛ Serving size: 1 oz (28.35 g); GI= 27 (Low); GL= 0.2 (Low); Net carb= 0.7 g

Queso—Fresco ☛ Serving size: 1 oz (28.35 g); GI= 27 (Low); GL= 0.5 (Low); Net carb= 1.9 g

Soy Cheese ☛ Serving size: 1 oz (28.35 g); GI= 40 (Low); GL= 2.7 (Low); Net carb= 6.8 g

Traditional Greek yoghurt ☛ Serving size: 1 cup (245 g); GI= 0.0 (Low); GL= 0 (Low); Net carb= 0 g

Yoghurt—lactose free ☛ Serving size: 1 cup (245 g); GI= 50 (Low); GL= 4.9 (Low); Net carb= 9.8 g

Yoghurt—natural low-fat ☛ Serving size: 1 cup (245 g); GI= 50 (Low); GL= 4.9 (Low); Net carb= 9.8 g

Yoghurt—natural regular-fat ☛ Serving size: 1 cup (245 g); GI= 50 (Low); GL= 4.9 (Low); Net carb= 9.8 g

Yogurt—chocolate, nonfat milk ☛ Serving size: 1 cup (245 g); GI= 32 (Low); GL= 3.1 (Low); Net carb= 9.7 g

Yogurt—frozen, chocolate, lowfat milk ☛ Serving size: 1 cup (245 g); GI= 50 (Low); GL= 4.9 (Low); Net carb= 9.8 g

Yogurt—frozen, chocolate, nonfat milk ☛ Serving size: 1 cup (245 g); GI= 50 (Low); GL= 4.9 (Low); Net carb= 9.8 g

Yogurt—frozen, chocolate, nonfat milk, with low-calorie sweetener ☛ Serving size: 1 cup (245 g); GI= 50 (Low); GL= 4.9 (Low); Net carb= 9.8 g

Yogurt—frozen, chocolate, whole milk ☛ Serving size: 1 cup (245 g); GI= 50 (Low); GL= 4.9 (Low); Net carb= 9.8 g

Yogurt—frozen, flavors other than chocolate, lowfat milk ☛ Serving size: 1 cup (245 g); GI= 50 (Low); GL= 4.9 (Low); Net carb= 9.8 g

Yogurt—frozen, flavors other than chocolate, nonfat milk ☛ Serving size: 1 cup (245 g); GI= 50 (Low); GL= 4.9 (Low); Net carb= 9.8 g

Yogurt—frozen, flavors other than chocolate, nonfat milk, with low-calorie sweetener ☛ Serving size: 1 cup (245 g); GI= 50 (Low); GL= 4.9 (Low); Net carb= 9.8 g

Yogurt—frozen, flavors other than chocolate, whole milk ☛ Serving size: 1 cup (245 g); GI= 50 (Low); GL= 4.9 (Low); Net carb= 9.8 g

Yogurt—frozen, flavors other than chocolate, with sorbet or sorbet-coated ☛ Serving size: 1 cup (245 g); GI= 50 (Low); GL= 4.9 (Low); Net carb= 9.8 g

Yogurt—fruit variety, lowfat milk ☛ Serving size: 1 cup (245 g); GI= 31 (Low); GL= 3 (Low); Net carb= 9.7 g

Yogurt—fruit variety, nonfat milk ☛ Serving size: 1 cup (245 g); GI= 32 (Low); GL= 3.1 (Low); Net carb= 9.7 g

Yogurt—fruit variety, nonfat milk, sweetened with low-calorie sweetener ☛ Serving size: 1 cup (245 g); GI= 19 (Low); GL= 1.9 (Low); Net carb= 10 g

Yogurt—fruit variety, whole milk ☛ Serving size: 1 cup (245 g); GI= 33 (Low); GL= 3.2 (Low); Net carb= 9.7 g

Yogurt—plain, lowfat milk ☛ Serving size: 1 cup (245 g); GI= 36 (Low); GL= 3.5 (Low); Net carb= 9.7 g

Yogurt—plain, nonfat milk ☛ Serving size: 1 cup (245 g); GI= 36 (Low); GL= 3.5 (Low); Net carb= 9.7 g

Yogurt—plain, whole milk ☛ Serving size: 1 cup (245 g); GI= 36 (Low); GL= 3.5 (Low); Net carb= 9.7 g

Yogurt—vanilla, lemon, maple, or coffee flavor, lowfat milk ☛ Serving size: 1 cup (245 g); GI= 27 (Low); GL= 2.6 (Low); Net carb= 9.6 g

Yogurt—vanilla, lemon, maple, or coffee flavor, nonfat milk ☛ Serving size: 1 cup (245 g); GI= 32 (Low); GL= 3.1 (Low); Net carb= 9.7 g

Yogurt—vanilla, lemon, maple, or coffee flavor, nonfat milk, sweetened with low-calorie sweetener ☛ Serving size: 1 cup (245 g); GI= 19 (Low); GL= 1.9 (Low); Net carb= 10 g

Yogurt—vanilla, lemon, or coffee flavor, whole milk ☛ Serving size: 1 cup (245 g); GI= 27 (Low); GL= 2.6 (Low); Net carb= 9.6 g

31
LEGUMS AND BEANS

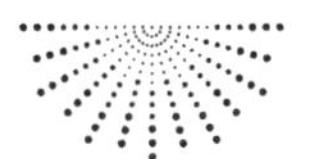

Adzuki Beans ☛ Serving size= ½ cup, 150 g; GI= 33 (Low); GL= 8.6 (Low); Net carb= 26.2 g

Baked Beans ☛ Serving size= ½ cup, 150 g; GI= 40 (Low); GL= 9.7 (Low); Net carb= 24.2 g

Bayo Beans—Canned Drained (cooked without fat) ☛ Serving size= ½ cup, 150 g; GI= 30 (Low); GL= 6.4 (Low); Net carb= 21.4 g

Bayo Beans—Canned Drained Made With Animal Fat Or Meat Drippings ☛ Serving size= ½ cup, 150 g; GI= 30 (Low); GL= 5.9 (Low); Net carb= 19.8 g

Bayo Beans—Canned Drained Made With Oil ☛ Serving size= ½ cup, 150 g; GI= 30 (Low); GL= 5.9 (Low); Net carb= 19.8 g

Bayo Beans—Dry Cooked (cooked without fat) ☛ Serving size= ½ cup, 150 g; GI= 30 (Low); GL= 6.7 (Low); Net carb= 22.3 g

Bayo Beans—Dry Cooked Made With Animal Fat Or Meat Drippings ☛ Serving size= ½ cup, 150 g; GI= 30 (Low); GL= 6.3 (Low); Net carb= 20.9 g

Bayo Beans—Dry Cooked Made With Oil ☛ Serving size= ½ cup, 150 g; GI= 30 (Low); GL= 6.2 (Low); Net carb= 20.8 g

Beans Adzuki—Mature Seed Cooked ☛ Serving size= ½ cup, 150 g; GI= 33 (Low); GL= 8.6 (Low); Net carb= 26.2 g

Beans Baked—Canned No Added Sugar ☛ Serving size= ½ cup, 150 g; GI= 40 (Low); GL= 9 (Low); Net carb= 22.5 g

Beans Baked—Canned With Franks ☛ Serving size= ½ cup, 150 g; GI= 40 (Low); GL= 5.1 (Low); Net carb= 12.7 g

Beans Baked—Canned With Pork ☛ Serving size= ½ cup, 150 g; GI= 40 (Low); GL= 8.7 (Low); Net carb= 21.7 g

Beans Baked—Canned With Pork And Tomato Sauce ☛ Serving size= ½ cup, 150 g; GI= 40 (Low); GL= 8.8 (Low); Net carb= 22 g

Black Beans—Mature Seeds Cooked ☛ Serving size= ½ cup, 150 g; GI= 30 (Low); GL= 6.8 (Low); Net carb= 22.5 g

Black Beans—Turtle Mature Seeds Canned ☛ Serving size= ½ cup, 150 g; GI= 41 (Low); GL= 5.9 (Low); Net carb= 14.5 g

Black Beans—Turtle Mature Seeds Cooked ☛ Serving size= ½ cup, 150 g; GI= 41 (Low); GL= 9.9 (Low); Net carb= 24.1 g

Broad Beans (Fava) ☛ Serving size= ½ cup, 150 g; GI= 40 (Low); GL= 8.6 (Low); Net carb= 21.4 g

Broad beans (Fava)—Mature Seeds Canned ☛ Serving size= ½ cup, 150 g; GI= 40 (Low); GL= 5.2 (Low); Net carb= 13.1 g

Broad beans (Fava)—Mature Seeds Cooked ☛ Serving size= ½ cup, 150 g; GI= 40 (Low); GL= 8.6 (Low); Net carb= 21.4 g

California Red Kidney Beans ☛ Serving size= ½ cup, 150 g; GI= 33 (Low); GL= 6.5 (Low); Net carb= 19.7 g

Chickpeas (Garbanzo)—Canned Drained (cooked without fat) ☛

Serving size= ½ cup, 150 g; GI= 36 (Low); GL= 8.2 (Low); Net carb= 22.7 g

Chickpeas (Garbanzo)—Canned Drained Made With Oil ☛ Serving size= ½ cup, 150 g; GI= 36 (Low); GL= 7.6 (Low); Net carb= 21.1 g

Chickpeas (Garbanzo)—Dry Cooked Made With Animal Fat Or Meat Drippings ☛ Serving size= ½ cup, 150 g; GI= 36 (Low); GL= 9.9 (Low); Net carb= 27.4 g

Chickpeas (Garbanzo)—Dry Cooked Made With Oil ☛ Serving size= ½ cup, 150 g; GI= 36 (Low); GL= 9.8 (Low); Net carb= 27.3 g

Chickpeas (Garbanzo)—Mature Seeds Canned Drained Rinsed In Tap Water ☛ Serving size= ½ cup, 150 g; GI= 36 (Low); GL= 8.9 (Low); Net carb= 24.9 g

Chickpeas (Garbanzo)—Mature Seeds Canned Drained Solids ☛ Serving size= ½ cup, 150 g; GI= 36 (Low); GL= 8.7 (Low); Net carb= 24.2 g

Chickpeas (Garbanzo)—Mature Seeds Canned Solids And Liquids ☛ Serving size= ½ cup, 150 g; GI= 36 (Low); GL= 4.9 (Low); Net carb= 13.6 g

Chickpeas (Garbanzo)—Stewed With Pig's Feet Puerto Rican Style ☛ Serving size= ½ cup, 150 g; GI= 36 (Low); GL= 3.6 (Low); Net carb= 9.9 g

Cowpeas—Dry Cooked (cooked with fat) ☛ Serving size= ½ cup, 150 g; GI= 50 (Low); GL= 9.8 (Low); Net carb= 19.7 g

Cowpeas—Mature Seeds Canned Plain ☛ Serving size= ½ cup, 150 g; GI= 50 (Low); GL= 7.7 (Low); Net carb= 15.5 g

Cowpeas—Mature Seeds Canned With Pork ☛ Serving size= ½ cup, 150 g; GI= 50 (Low); GL= 9.9 (Low); Net carb= 19.8 g

Edamame ☛ Serving size= ½ cup, 150 g; GI= 20 (Low); GL= 1.1 (Low); Net carb= 5.6 g

Extra Firm Tofu ☛ Serving size= ½ cup, 150 g; GI= 15 (Low); GL= 0.2 (Low); Net carb= 1.2 g

French Beans—Mature Seeds Cooked ☛ Serving size= ½ cup, 150 g; GI= 21 (Low); GL= 4.6 (Low); Net carb= 21.9 g

French Beans—Mature Seeds Cooked Boiled Without Salt ☛ Serving size= ½ cup, 150 g; GI= 21 (Low); GL= 4.6 (Low); Net carb= 21.9 g

Green Or Yellow Split Peas—Dry Cooked (cooked without fat) ☛ Serving size= ½ cup, 150 g; GI= 33 (Low); GL= 6.3 (Low); Net carb= 19 g

Green Or Yellow Split Peas—Dry Cooked Made With Animal Fat Or Meat Drippings ☛ Serving size= ½ cup, 150 g; GI= 33 (Low); GL= 5.9 (Low); Net carb= 17.9 g

Green Or Yellow Split Peas—Dry Cooked Made With Oil ☛ Serving size= ½ cup, 150 g; GI= 33 (Low); GL= 5.9 (Low); Net carb= 17.9 g

Green Soybeans ☛ Serving size= ½ cup, 150 g; GI= 18 (Low); GL= 1.8 (Low); Net carb= 10.3 g

Hummus (Commercial) ☛ Serving size= 1 tbsp, 15 g; GI= 15 (Low); GL= 0.2 (Low); Net carb= 1.4 g

Hummus (Homemade) ☛ Serving size= 1 tbsp, 15 g; GI= 15 (Low); GL= 0.4 (Low); Net carb= 2.4 g

Kidney Beans ☛ Serving size= ½ cup, 150 g; GI= 33 (Low); GL= 8.1 (Low); Net carb= 24.6 g

Kidney Beans—All Types Mature Seeds Cooked ☛ Serving size= ½ cup, 150 g; GI= 34 (Low); GL= 8.4 (Low); Net carb= 24.6 g

Kidney Beans—California Red Mature Seeds Cooked ☛ Serving size= ½ cup, 150 g; GI= 34 (Low); GL= 6.7 (Low); Net carb= 19.7 g

Kidney Beans—Red Mature Seeds Cooked ☛ Serving size= ½ cup, 150 g; GI= 33 (Low); GL= 7.6 (Low); Net carb= 23.1 g

Kidney Beans—Royal Red Mature Seeds Cooked ☛ Serving size= ½ cup, 150 g; GI= 33 (Low); GL= 6.2 (Low); Net carb= 18.8 g

Lentils (Cooked) ☛ Serving size= ½ cup, 150 g; GI= 21 (Low); GL= 3.9 (Low); Net carb= 18.3 g

Lentils—Dry Cooked (cooked without fat) ☛ Serving size= ½ cup, 150 g; GI= 21 (Low); GL= 3.8 (Low); Net carb= 18.2 g

Lentils—Dry Cooked Made With Animal Fat Or Meat Drippings ☛ Serving size= ½ cup, 150 g; GI= 21 (Low); GL= 3.6 (Low); Net carb= 17.1 g

Lentils—Dry Cooked Made With Oil ☛ Serving size= ½ cup, 150 g; GI= 21 (Low); GL= 3.6 (Low); Net carb= 17 g

Lentils—Mature Seeds Cooked ☛ Serving size= ½ cup, 150 g; GI= 21 (Low); GL= 3.7 (Low); Net carb= 17.5 g

Lima Beans ☛ Serving size= ½ cup, 150 g; GI= 46 (Low); GL= 9.6 (Low); Net carb= 20.8 g

Lima Beans—Dry Cooked (cooked without fat) ☛ Serving size= ½ cup, 150 g; GI= 46 (Low); GL= 9.5 (Low); Net carb= 20.7 g

Lima Beans—Dry Cooked Made With Animal Fat Or Meat Drippings ☛ Serving size= ½ cup, 150 g; GI= 46 (Low); GL= 8.9 (Low); Net carb= 19.4 g

Lima Beans—Dry Cooked Made With Oil ☛ Serving size= ½ cup, 150 g; GI= 46 (Low); GL= 8.9 (Low); Net carb= 19.3 g

Lima Beans—Large Mature Seeds Cooked ☛ Serving size= ½ cup, 150 g; GI= 46 (Low); GL= 9.6 (Low); Net carb= 20.8 g

Miso ☛ Serving size= 1 tbsp, 17 g; GI= 63 (Medium); GL= 2.1 (Low); Net carb= 3.4 g

Mung Beans (Cooked) ☛ Serving size= ½ cup, 150 g; GI= 42 (Low); GL= 7.3 (Low); Net carb= 17.3 g

Mung Beans—Dry Cooked (cooked with fat) ☛ Serving size= ½ cup, 150 g; GI= 42 (Low); GL= 6.8 (Low); Net carb= 16.1 g

Mung Beans—Dry Cooked (cooked without fat) ☛ Serving size= ½ cup, 150 g; GI= 42 (Low); GL= 7.2 (Low); Net carb= 17.2 g

Mung Beans—Mature Seeds Cooked ☛ Serving size= ½ cup, 150 g; GI= 42 (Low); GL= 7.3 (Low); Net carb= 17.3 g

Natto ☛ Serving size= ½ cup, 150 g; GI= 54 (Low); GL= 5.9 (Low); Net carb= 10.9 g

Navy Beans ☛ Serving size= ½ cup, 150 g; GI= 39 (Low); GL= 9.1 (Low); Net carb= 23.3 g

Navy Beans—Mature Seeds Cooked ☛ Serving size= ½ cup, 150 g; GI= 39 (Low); GL= 9.1 (Low); Net carb= 23.3 g

Okara ☛ Serving size= 1 cup, 122 g; GI= 53 (Low); GL= 7.9 (Low); Net carb= 14.9 g

Peanut Butter (Chunk Style) ☛ Serving size= 2 tbsp, 32 g; GI= 14 (Low); GL= 0.6 (Low); Net carb= 4.3 g

Peanut Butter (Smooth) ☛ Serving size= 2 tbsp, 32 g; GI= 14 (Low); GL= 0.8 (Low); Net carb= 5.8 g

Peanut Spread Reduced Sugar ☛ Serving size= 2 tbsp, 31 g; GI= 14 (Low); GL= 0.3 (Low); Net carb= 2 g

Peanuts—Spanish Raw ☛ Serving size= 1 cup, 146 g; GI= 13 (Low); GL= 1.2 (Low); Net carb= 9.2 g

Peanuts—Valencia Oil-Roasted With Salt ☛ Serving size= 1 cup, 144 g; GI= 13 (Low); GL= 1.4 (Low); Net carb= 10.7 g

Peanuts—Valencia Oil-Roasted Without Salt ☛ Serving size= 1 cup, 144 g; GI= 13 (Low); GL= 1.4 (Low); Net carb= 10.7 g

Peanuts—Valencia Raw ☛ Serving size= 1 cup, 146 g; GI= 13 (Low); GL= 2.3 (Low); Net carb= 17.8 g

Peas—Dry Cooked With Pork ☛ Serving size= ½ cup, 150 g; GI= 22 (Low); GL= 3.5 (Low); Net carb= 16 g

Peas—Split Mature Seeds Cooked ☛ Serving size= ½ cup, 150 g; GI= 51 (Low); GL= 9.3 (Low); Net carb= 18.3 g

Pigeon Peas—Mature Seeds Cooked ☛ Serving size= ½ cup, 150 g; GI= 31 (Low); GL= 7.7 (Low); Net carb= 24.8 g

Pigeon Peas—Mature Seeds Cooked Boiled Without Salt ☛ Serving size= ½ cup, 150 g; GI= 31 (Low); GL= 7.7 (Low); Net carb= 24.8 g

Pinto Beans—Canned Drained Solids ☛ Serving size= ½ cup, 150 g; GI= 39 (Low); GL= 8.6 (Low); Net carb= 22.1 g

Pinto Beans—Mature Seeds Canned Solids And Liquids ☛ Serving size= ½ cup, 150 g; GI= 39 (Low); GL= 6.2 (Low); Net carb= 15.9 g

Red Kidney Beans—Canned Drained (cooked without fat) ☛ Serving size= ½ cup, 150 g; GI= 35 (Low); GL= 8.8 (Low); Net carb= 25.1 g

Red Kidney Beans—Canned Drained Made With Oil ☛ Serving size= ½ cup, 150 g; GI= 35 (Low); GL= 8.2 (Low); Net carb= 23.4 g

Red Kidney Beans—Dry Cooked (cooked without fat) ☛ Serving size= ½ cup, 150 g; GI= 35 (Low); GL= 8 (Low); Net carb= 22.9 g

Red Kidney Beans—Dry Cooked Made With Animal Fat Or Meat Drippings ☛ Serving size= ½ cup, 150 g; GI= 35 (Low); GL= 7.5 (Low); Net carb= 21.4 g

Red Kidney Beans—Dry Cooked Made With Oil ☛ Serving size= ½ cup, 150 g; GI= 35 (Low); GL= 7.5 (Low); Net carb= 21.4 g

Silk (Soy Milk) ☛ Serving size= 1 cup, 243 g; GI= 30 (Low); GL= 2.1 (Low); Net carb= 7 g

Silk Chai Soy Milk ☛ Serving size= 1 cup, 243 g; GI= 30 (Low); GL= 5.7 (Low); Net carb= 19 g

Silk Chocolate Soy Milk ☛ Serving size= 1 cup, 243 g; GI= 30 (Low); GL= 6.3 (Low); Net carb= 21.1 g

Silk Plus Fiber Soy Milk ☛ Serving size= 1 cup, 243 g; GI= 30 (Low); GL= 2.7 (Low); Net carb= 8.9 g

Silk Plus For Bone Health Soy Milk ☛ Serving size= 1 cup, 243 g; GI= 30 (Low); GL= 2.7 (Low); Net carb= 9.1 g

Silk Plus Omega-3 Dha Soy Milk ☛ Serving size= 1 cup, 243 g; GI= 30 (Low); GL= 2.1 (Low); Net carb= 7 g

Silk Vanilla Soy Milk ☛ Serving size= 1 cup, 243 g; GI= 30 (Low); GL= 2.7 (Low); Net carb= 9 g

Small White Beans—Mature Seeds Cooked ☛ Serving size= ½ cup, 150 g; GI= 36 (Low); GL= 8.3 (Low); Net carb= 23.1 g

Soft Tofu ☛ Serving size= 1 piece (2 1/2 inch * 2 3/4 inch * 1 inch), 120 g; GI= 15 (Low); GL= 0.2 (Low); Net carb= 1.2 g

Soy Flour—Defatted ☛ Serving size= 1 cup, 105 g; GI= 25 (Low); GL= 4.3 (Low); Net carb= 17.2 g

Soy Flour—Full-Fat Raw ☛ Serving size= 1 cup, stirred, 84 g; GI= 25 (Low); GL= 4.7 (Low); Net carb= 18.7 g

Soy Flour—Full-Fat Roasted ☛ Serving size= 1 cup, stirred, 85 g; GI= 25 (Low); GL= 4.4 (Low); Net carb= 17.6 g

Soy Milk ☛ Serving size= 1 cup, 243 g; GI= 30 (Low); GL= 0.9 (Low); Net carb= 3 g

Soy Milk (All Flavors) Enhanced ☛ Serving size= 1 cup, 243 g; GI= 30 (Low); GL= 2.2 (Low); Net carb= 7.4 g

Soy Protein—Concentrate Made By Acid Wash ☛ Serving size= 1 oz, 28.4 g; GI= 47 (Low); GL= 2.7 (Low); Net carb= 5.7 g

Soy Protein—Concentrate Made By Alcohol Extraction ☛ Serving size= 1 oz, 28.4 g; GI= 47 (Low); GL= 2.7 (Low); Net carb= 5.7 g

Soy Protein—Isolate Potassium Type ☛ Serving size= 1 oz, 28.4 g; GI= 47 (Low); GL= 0.3 (Low); Net carb= 0.7 g

Soy Protein—Powder (Isolate) ☛ Serving size= 1 oz, 28.4 g; GI= 47 (Low); GL= 0 (Low); Net carb= 0 g

Soy Sauce without added sugar ☛ Serving size= 1 tbsp, 16 g; GI= 20 (Low); GL= 0.1 (Low); Net carb= 0.7 g

Soybean Curd ☛ Serving size= 1 slice (2 3/4" * 1" * 1/2"), 29 g; GI= 15 (Low); GL= 0.3 (Low); Net carb= 2.3 g

Soybeans—Dry Cooked (cooked with fat) ☛ Serving size= 1 cup, 180 g; GI= 31 (Low); GL= 1.2 (Low); Net carb= 4 g

Soybeans—Dry Cooked (cooked without fat) ☛ Serving size= 1 cup, 180 g; GI= 31 (Low); GL= 1.3 (Low); Net carb= 4.2 g

Soybeans—Mature Seeds Cooked ☛ Serving size= 1 cup, 172 g; GI= 31 (Low); GL= 1.3 (Low); Net carb= 4.1 g

Tamari, without added sugar ☛ Serving size= 1 tbsp, 18 g; GI= 20 (Low); GL= 0.2 (Low); Net carb= 0.9 g

Tempeh ☛ Serving size= 1 cup, 166 g; GI= 15 (Low); GL= 1.9 (Low); Net carb= 12.7 g

Tofu Silken Extra Firm ☛ Serving size= 1 slice, 84 g; GI= 15 (Low); GL= 0.2 (Low); Net carb= 1.6 g

Tofu Silken Firm ☛ Serving size= 1 slice, 84 g; GI= 15 (Low); GL= 0.3 (Low); Net carb= 1.9 g

Unsweetened Soy Milk ☛ Serving size= 1 cup, 243 g; GI= 30 (Low); GL= 0.9 (Low); Net carb= 3 g

White Beans—Mature Seeds Canned ☛ Serving size= ½ cup, 150 g; GI= 36 (Low); GL= 8.9 (Low); Net carb= 24.6 g

Yellow Beans—Mature Seeds Cooked ☛ Serving size= ½ cup, 150 g; GI= 36 (Low); GL= 8 (Low); Net carb= 22.3 g

Yellow Beans—Mature Seeds Cooked Boiled Without Salt ☛ Serving size= ½ cup, 150 g; GI= 36 (Low); GL= 8 (Low); Net carb= 22.3 g

32

FISH & FISH PRODUCTS

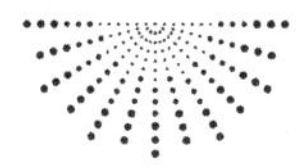

Anchovy—canned, oil or water ☛ Serving size= 3 0z (85 g); GI= 0 (Low); GL= 0 (Low)

Carp—baked or broiled ☛ Serving size= 3 0z (85 g); GI= 50 (Low); GL= 1 (Low)

Carp—floured or breaded, fried ☛ Serving size= 3 0z (85 g); GI= 95 (High); GL= 7.8 (Low)

Carp—steamed or poached ☛ Serving size= 3 0z (85 g); GI= 0 (Low); GL= 0 (Low)

Catfish—baked or broiled ☛ Serving size= 1 fillet (150 g); GI= 50 (Low); GL= 1 (Low)

Catfish—battered, fried ☛ Serving size= 1 fillet (150 g); GI= 95 (High); GL= 7.8 (Low)

Catfish—breaded or battered, baked ☛ Serving size= 1 fillet (150 g); GI= 95 (High); GL= 7.8 (Low)

Catfish—floured or breaded, fried ☛ Serving size= 1 fillet (150 g); GI= 95 (High); GL= 7.8 (Low)

Catfish—steamed or poached ☛ Serving size= 1 fillet (150 g); GI= 0 (Low); GL= 0 (Low)

Clams—baked or broiled ☛ Serving size= 3 0z (85 g); GI= 50 (Low); GL= 1.8 (Low)

Clams—canned, oil or water ☛ Serving size= 3 0z (85 g); GI= 50 (Low); GL= 1.8 (Low)

Clams—raw ☛ Serving size= 3 0z (85 g); GI= 50 (Low); GL= 1.8 (Low)

Clams—steamed or boiled ☛ Serving size= 3 0z (85 g); GI= 50 (Low); GL= 1.8 (Low)

Cod—baked or broiled ☛ Serving size= 3 0z (85 g); GI= 50 (Low); GL= 1.1 (Low)

Cod—battered, fried ☛ Serving size= 3 0z (85 g); GI= 95 (High); GL= 7.8 (Low)

Cod—breaded or battered, baked ☛ Serving size= 3 0z (85 g); GI= 95 (High); GL= 7.8 (Low)

Cod—floured or breaded, fried ☛ Serving size= 3 0z (85 g); GI= 95 (High); GL= 7.8 (Low)

Cod—steamed or poached ☛ Serving size= 3 0z (85 g); GI= 0 (Low); GL= 0 (Low)

Conch—baked or broiled ☛ Serving size= 3 0z (85 g); GI= 50 (Low); GL= 1.3 (Low)

Crab—baked or broiled ☛ Serving size= 3 0z (85 g); GI= 50 (Low); GL= 1.2 (Low)

Crab—hard shell, steamed ☛ Serving size= 3 0z (85 g); GI= 0 (Low); GL= 0 (Low)

Crayfish—floured, fried ☛ Serving size= 3 0z (85 g); GI= 95 (High); GL= 7.8 (Low)

Croaker—baked or broiled ☛ Serving size= 3 0z (85 g); GI= 50 (Low); GL= 1 (Low)

Croaker—floured or breaded, fried ☛ Serving size= 3 0z (85 g); GI= 95 (High); GL= 7.8 (Low)

Croaker—steamed or poached ☛ Serving size= 3 0z (85 g); GI= 0 (Low); GL= 0 (Low)

Fish, in general—baked or broiled ☛ Serving size= 3 0z (85 g); GI= 50 (Low); GL= 1 (Low)

Fish, in general—battered, fried ☛ Serving size= 3 0z (85 g); GI= 95 (High); GL= 7.8 (Low)

Fish, in general—breaded or battered, baked ☛ Serving size= 3 0z (85 g); GI= 95 (High); GL= 7.8 (Low)

Fish, in general—canned ☛ Serving size= 3 0z (85 g); GI= 0 (Low); GL= 0 (Low)

Fish, in general—floured or breaded, fried ☛ Serving size= 3 0z (85 g); GI= 95 (High); GL= 7.8 (Low)

Fish, in general—smoked ☛ Serving size= 1 oz; GI= 0 (Low); GL= 0 (Low)

Fish, in general—steamed ☛ Serving size= 3 0z (85 g); GI= 0 (Low); GL= 0 (Low)

Flounder—baked or broiled ☛ Serving size= 3 0z (85 g); GI= 50 (Low); GL= 1 (Low)

Flounder—battered, fried ☛ Serving size= 3 0z (85 g); GI= 95 (High); GL= 7.8 (Low)

Flounder—breaded or battered, baked ☛ Serving size= 3 0z (85 g); GI= 95 (High); GL= 7.8 (Low)

Flounder—floured or breaded, fried ☛ Serving size= 3 0z (85 g); GI= 95 (High); GL= 7.8 (Low)

Flounder—steamed or poached ☛ Serving size= 3 0z (85 g); GI= 0 (Low); GL= 0 (Low)

Haddock—baked or broiled ☛ Serving size= 3 0z (85 g); GI= 50 (Low); GL= 1.1 (Low)

Haddock—battered, fried ☛ Serving size= 3 0z (85 g); GI= 95 (High); GL= 7.8 (Low)

Haddock—breaded or battered, baked ☛ Serving size= 3 0z (85 g); GI= 95 (High); GL= 7.8 (Low)

Haddock—floured or breaded, fried ☛ Serving size= 3 0z (85 g); GI= 95 (High); GL= 7.8 (Low)

Haddock—steamed or poached ☛ Serving size= 3 0z (85 g); GI= 0 (Low); GL= 1 (Low)

Herring—baked or broiled ☛ Serving size= 1 fillet (150 g); GI= 50 (Low); GL= 1.1 (Low)

Herring—pickled ☛ Serving size= 1 fillet (150 g); GI= 50 (Low); GL= 1.1 (Low)

Herring—raw ☛ Serving size= 1 fillet (150 g); GI= 0 (Low); GL= 0 (Low)

Herring—smoked, kippered ☛ Serving size= 1 oz; GI= 0 (Low); GL= 0 (Low)

Lobster—baked or broiled ☛ Serving size= 3 0z (85 g); GI= 50 (Low); GL= 1.9 (Low)

Lobster—steamed or boiled ☛ Serving size= 3 0z (85 g); GI= 50 (Low); GL= 1.9 (Low)

Lobster—without shell, steamed or boiled ☛ Serving size= 3 0z (85 g); GI= 50 (Low); GL= 1.9 (Low)

Mackerel—baked or broiled ☛ Serving size= 3 0z (85 g); GI= 50 (Low); GL= 1 (Low)

Mackerel—canned ☛ Serving size= 3 0z (85 g); GI= 0 (Low); GL= 0 (Low)

Mackerel—floured or breaded, fried ☛ Serving size= 3 0z (85 g); GI= 95 (High); GL= 7.8 (Low)

Mullet—baked or broiled ☛ Serving size= 1 fillet (150 g); GI= 50 (Low); GL= 1.1 (Low)

Mullet—floured or breaded, fried ☛ Serving size= 1 fillet (150 g); GI= 95 (High); GL= 7.8 (Low)

Mussels—steamed or poached ☛ Serving size= 3 0z (85 g); GI= 50 (Low); GL= 1.1 (Low)

Ocean perch—baked or broiled ☛ Serving size= 1 fillet (150 g); GI= 50 (Low); GL= 1.1 (Low)

Ocean perch—battered, fried ☛ Serving size= 1 fillet (150 g); GI= 95 (High); GL= 7.8 (Low)

Ocean perch—breaded or battered, baked ☛ Serving size= 1 fillet (150 g); GI= 95 (High); GL= 7.8 (Low)

Ocean perch—floured or breaded, fried ☛ Serving size= 1 fillet (150 g); GI= 95 (High); GL= 7.8 (Low)

Ocean perch—raw ☛ Serving size= 1 fillet (150 g); GI= 0 (Low); GL= 0 (Low)

Octopus—dried, boiled ☛ Serving size= 3 0z (85 g); GI= 50 (Low); GL= 1.1 (Low)

Oysters—baked or broiled ☛ Serving size= about 12 medium; GI= 50 (Low); GL= 1.1 (Low)

Oysters—canned ☛ Serving size= about 12 medium; GI= 50 (Low); GL= 1.1 (Low)

Oysters—raw ☛ Serving size= about 12 medium; GI= 50 (Low); GL= 1.1 (Low)

Oysters—smoked ☛ Serving size= 1 oz; GI= 50 (Low); GL= 1.1 (Low)

Perch—baked or broiled ☛ Serving size= 1 fillet (150 g); GI= 50 (Low); GL= 1.1 (Low)

Perch—battered, fried ☛ Serving size= 1 fillet (150 g); GI= 95 (High); GL= 7.8 (Low)

Perch—breaded or battered, baked ☛ Serving size= 1 fillet (150 g); GI= 95 (High); GL= 7.8 (Low)

Perch—floured or breaded, fried ☛ Serving size= 1 fillet (150 g); GI= 95 (High); GL= 7.8 (Low)

Perch—steamed or poached ☛ Serving size= 1 fillet (150 g); GI= 0 (Low); GL= 0 (Low)

Pike—baked or broiled ☛ Serving size= 1 fillet (150 g); GI= 50 (Low); GL= 1.1 (Low)

Pompano—baked or broiled ☛ Serving size= 1 fillet (150 g); GI= 50 (Low); GL= 1.1 (Low)

Pompano—floured or breaded, fried ☛ Serving size= 1 fillet (150 g); GI= 95 (High); GL= 7.8 (Low)

Pompano—raw ☛ Serving size= 1 fillet (150 g); GI= 0 (Low); GL= 0 (Low)

Porgy—baked or broiled ☛ Serving size= 1 fillet (150 g); GI= 50 (Low); GL= 1.1 (Low)

Porgy—battered, fried ☛ Serving size= 1 fillet (150 g); GI= 95 (High); GL= 7.8 (Low)

Porgy—breaded or battered, baked ☛ Serving size= 1 fillet (150 g); GI= 95 (High); GL= 7.8 (Low)

Porgy—floured or breaded, fried ☛ Serving size= 1 fillet (150 g); GI= 95 (High); GL= 7.8 (Low)

Porgy—raw ☛ Serving size= 1 fillet (150 g); GI= 0 (Low); GL= 0 (Low)

Porgy—steamed or poached ☛ Serving size= 1 fillet (150 g); GI= 0 (Low); GL= 0 (Low)

Roe—cooked ☛ Serving size= 1 oz; GI= 50 (Low); GL= 1.1 (Low)

Roe—sturgeon ☛ Serving size= 1 oz; GI= 50 (Low); GL= 1.1 (Low)

Salmon—baked or broiled ☛ Serving size= 1 fillet (150 g); GI= 50 (Low); GL= 1.1 (Low)

Salmon—battered, fried ☛ Serving size= 1 fillet (150 g); GI= 95 (High); GL= 7.8 (Low)

Salmon—canned, oil or water ☛ Serving size= 1 fillet (150 g); GI= 0 (Low); GL= 0 (Low)

Salmon—floured or breaded, fried ☛ Serving size= 1 fillet (150 g); GI= 95 (High); GL= 7.8 (Low)

Salmon—smoked ☛ Serving size= 1 oz; GI= 0 (Low); GL= 0 (Low)

Salmon—steamed or poached ☛ Serving size= 1 fillet (150 g); GI= 0 (Low); GL= 0 (Low)

Sardines—canned in oil ☛ Serving size= 3 0z (85 g); GI= 0 (Low); GL= 0 (Low)

Sardines—cooked ☛ Serving size= 6 0z (170 g); GI= 0 (Low); GL= 0 (Low)

Sardines—skinless, boneless, canned in water or oil ☛ Serving size= 6 0z (170 g); GI= 0 (Low); GL= 0 (Low)

Scallops—baked or broiled ☛ Serving size= about

6 large

or 14 small; GI= 50 (Low); GL= 1.9 (Low)

Scallops—steamed or boiled ☛ Serving size= about

6 large

or 14 small; GI= 50 (Low); GL= 1.9 (Low)

Sea bass—baked or broiled ☛ Serving size= 1 fillet (150 g); GI= 50 (Low); GL= 1 (Low)

Sea bass—floured or breaded, fried ☛ Serving size= 1 fillet (150 g); GI= 95 (High); GL= 8.2 (Low)

Sea bass—steamed or poached ☛ Serving size= 1 fillet (150 g); GI= 0 (Low); GL= 0 (Low)

Shark—steamed or poached ☛ Serving size= 6 0z (170 g); GI= 0 (Low); GL= 0 (Low)

Shrimp—baked or broiled ☛ Serving size= 3 0z (85 g); GI= 50 (Low); GL= 1.8 (Low)

Shrimp—canned, oil or water ☛ Serving size= 3 0z (85 g); GI= 50 (Low); GL= 1.8 (Low)

Shrimp—floured, fried ☛ Serving size= 3 0z (85 g); GI= 95 (High); GL= 8.2 (Low)

Shrimp—steamed or boiled ☛ Serving size= 3 0z (85 g); GI= 50 (Low); GL= 1.8 (Low)

Smelt—battered, fried ☛ Serving size= 6 0z (170 g); GI= 95 (High); GL= 7.8 (Low)

Smelt—floured or breaded, fried ☛ Serving size= 6 0z (170 g); GI= 95 (High); GL= 7.8 (Low)

Squid—baked, broiled ☛ Serving size= 6 0z (170 g); GI= 50 (Low); GL= 1.7 (Low)

Squid—breaded, fried ☛ Serving size= 6 0z (170 g); GI= 95 (High); GL= 7.8 (Low)

Squid—canned in oil or water ☛ Serving size= 6 0z (170 g); GI= 50 (Low); GL= 1.7 (Low)

Squid—pickled ☛ Serving size= 3 0z (85 g); GI= 50 (Low); GL= 1.7 (Low)

Squid—steamed or boiled ☛ Serving size= 6 0z (170 g); GI= 50 (Low); GL= 1.7 (Low)

Swordfish—baked or broiled ☛ Serving size= 6 0z (170 g); GI= 50 (Low); GL= 1 (Low)

Swordfish—floured or breaded, fried ☛ Serving size= 6 0z (170 g); GI= 95 (High); GL= 7.8 (Low)

Swordfish—steamed or poached ☛ Serving size= 6 0z (170 g); GI= 0 (Low); GL= 0 (Low)

Trout—baked or broiled ☛ Serving size= 1 fillet (150 g); GI= 50 (Low); GL= 1 (Low)

Trout—battered, fried ☛ Serving size= 1 fillet (150 g); GI= 95 (High); GL= 7.8 (Low)

Trout—breaded or battered, baked ☛ Serving size= 1 fillet (150 g); GI= 95 (High); GL= 7.8 (Low)

Trout—floured or breaded, fried ☛ Serving size= 1 fillet (150 g); GI= 95 (High); GL= 7.8 (Low)

Trout—smoked ☛ Serving size= 1 oz; GI= 0 (Low); GL= 0 (Low)

Trout—steamed or poached ☛ Serving size= 1 fillet (150 g); GI= 0 (Low); GL= 0 (Low)

Tuna—canned, in oil or water ☛ Serving size= 3 0z (85 g); GI= 0 (Low); GL= 0 (Low)

Tuna—canned, in oil ☛ Serving size= 3 0z (85 g); GI= 0 (Low); GL= 0 (Low)

Tuna—canned, in water ☛ Serving size= 3 0z (85 g); GI= 0 (Low); GL= 0 (Low)

Tuna—fresh—baked or broiled ☛ Serving size= 6 0z (170 g); GI= 50

(Low); GL= 1 (Low)

Tuna—fresh—floured or breaded, fried ☛ Serving size= 6 0z (170 g); GI= 95 (High); GL= 7.8 (Low)

Tuna—fresh—steamed or poached ☛ Serving size= 6 0z (170 g); GI= 0 (Low); GL= 0 (Low)

Tuna—fresh, raw ☛ Serving size= 6 0z (170 g); GI= 0 (Low); GL= 0 (Low)

Whiting—baked or broiled ☛ Serving size= 6 0z (170 g); GI= 50 (Low); GL= 1 (Low)

Whiting—battered, fried ☛ Serving size= 6 0z (170 g); GI= 95 (High); GL= 7.8 (Low)

Whiting—floured or breaded, fried ☛ Serving size= 6 0z (170 g); GI= 95 (High); GL= 7.8 (Low)

33
FRUITS AND FRUITS PRODUCTS

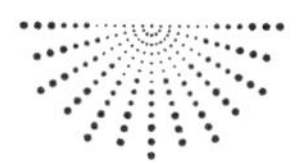

Apple Baked—unsweetened ☛ Serving size= 1 apple with liquid, 161 (g); GI= 38 (Low); GL= 7.5 (Low); Net carbs= 19.7 g

Apple Chips ☛ Serving size= 1 cup, 28 (g); GI= 35 (Low); GL= 6.3 (Low); Net carbs= 17.9 g

Apple Pickled ☛ Serving size= 1 apple, 29 (g); GI= 38 (Low); GL= 3.4 (Low); Net carbs= 8.8 g

Apple Rings Fried ☛ Serving size= 1 ring, 19 (g); GI= 38 (Low); GL= 1.2 (Low); Net carbs= 3.2 g

Apples ☛ Serving size= 1 cup, quartered or chopped, 125 (g); GI= 38 (Low); GL= 5.4 (Low); Net carbs= 14.3 g

Apples—(Without Skin) ☛ Serving size= 1 cup slices, 110 (g); GI= 41 (Low); GL= 5.2 (Low); Net carbs= 12.6 g

Apples—Frozen—unsweetened Heated ☛ Serving size= 1 cup slices, 206 (g); GI= 38 (Low); GL= 8.4 (Low); Net carbs= 22 g

Apples—Frozen—unsweetened Unheated ☛ Serving size= 1 cup slices, 173 (g); GI= 38 (Low); GL= 7.2 (Low); Net carbs= 19 g

Apples—Raw Without Skin Cooked Boiled ☛ Serving size= 1 cup slices, 171 (g); GI= 38 (Low); GL= 7.3 (Low); Net carbs= 19.2 g

Apples—Raw Without Skin Cooked Microwave ☛ Serving size= 1 cup slices, 170 (g); GI= 38 (Low); GL= 7.5 (Low); Net carbs= 19.7 g

Apricots ☛ Serving size= 1 cup, halves, 155 (g); GI= 31 (Low); GL= 4.4 (Low); Net carbs= 14.1 g

Asian Pears ☛ Serving size= 1 fruit 2-1/4 inch high x 2-1/2 inch dia, 122 (g); GI= 26 (Low); GL= 2.2 (Low); Net carbs= 8.6 g

Avocados ☛ Serving size= 1 cup, cubes, 150 (g); GI= 50 (Low); GL= 1.4 (Low); Net carbs= 2.7 g

Banana—Red Fried ☛ Serving size= 1 fruit (7-1/4" long), 94 (g); GI= 49 (Low); GL= 9.8 (Low); Net carbs= 20 g

Banana—Ripe Fried ☛ Serving size= 1 small, 73 (g); GI= 62 (Medium); GL= 9.6 (Low); Net carbs= 15.5 g

Bartlett Pears ☛ Serving size= 1 cup, sliced, 140 (g); GI= 41 (Low); GL= 6.8 (Low); Net carbs= 16.7 g

Blackberries ☛ Serving size= 1 cup, 144 (g); GI= 25 (Low); GL= 1.6 (Low); Net carbs= 6.2 g

Blackberries Frozen—unsweetened ☛ Serving size= 1 cup, unthawed, 151 (g); GI= 25 (Low); GL= 4 (Low); Net carbs= 16.1 g

Blueberries ☛ Serving size= 1 cup, 148 (g); GI= 53 (Low); GL= 9.5 (Low); Net carbs= 17.9 g

Blueberries (Frozen) ☛ Serving size= 1 cup, unthawed, 155 (g); GI= 53 (Low); GL= 7.8 (Low); Net carbs= 14.7 g

Bosc Pear ☛ Serving size= 1 cup, sliced, 140 (g); GI= 41 (Low); GL= 7.5 (Low); Net carbs= 18.2 g

Boysenberries (Frozen) ☛ Serving size= 1 cup, unthawed, 132 (g); GI= 43 (Low); GL= 3.9 (Low); Net carbs= 9.1 g

California Avocados ☛ Serving size= 1 cup, pureed, 230 (g); GI= 50 (Low); GL= 2.1 (Low); Net carbs= 4.2 g

California Grapefruit ☛ Serving size= 1 cup sections, with juice, 230 (g); GI= 25 (Low); GL= 5.6 (Low); Net carbs= 22.3 g

California Valencia Oranges ☛ Serving size= 1 cup sections, without membranes, 180 (g); GI= 42 (Low); GL= 7.1 (Low); Net carbs= 16.9 g

Cantaloupe Melons ☛ Serving size= 1 cup, balls, 177 (g); GI= 61 (Medium); GL= 7.8 (Low); Net carbs= 12.9 g

Casaba Melon ☛ Serving size= 1 cup, cubes, 170 (g); GI= 62 (Medium); GL= 6 (Low); Net carbs= 9.7 g

Cherries (Sweet) ☛ Serving size= 1 cup, with pits, yields, 138 (g); GI= 22 (Low); GL= 4.2 (Low); Net carbs= 19.2 g

Clementines ☛ Serving size= 1 fruit, 74 (g); GI= 35 (Low); GL= 2.7 (Low); Net carbs= 7.6 g

Cranberries ☛ Serving size= 1 cup, chopped, 110 (g); GI= 45 (Low); GL= 4.1 (Low); Net carbs= 9.2 g

Dried Litchis ☛ Serving size= 1 fruit, 2.5 (g); GI= 60 (Medium); GL= 1 (Low); Net carbs= 1.7 g

European Black Currants ☛ Serving size= 1 cup, 112 (g); GI= 22 (Low); GL= 3.8 (Low); Net carbs= 17.2 g

Figs ☛ Serving size= 1 large (2-1/2 inch dia), 64 (g); GI= 51 (Low); GL= 5.3 (Low); Net carbs= 10.4 g

Florida Avocados ☛ Serving size= 1 cup, pureed, 230 (g); GI= 50 (Low); GL= 2.6 (Low); Net carbs= 5.1 g

Florida Grapefruit ☛ Serving size= 1 cup sections, with juice, 230 (g); GI= 25 (Low); GL= 3.7 (Low); Net carbs= 14.7 g

Florida Oranges ☛ Serving size= 1 cup sections, without membranes, 185 (g); GI= 42 (Low); GL= 7.1 (Low); Net carbs= 16.9 g

Fruit Salad—Fresh Or Raw Including Citrus Fruits No Dressing ☛ Serving size= 1 cup, 175 (g); GI= 51 (Low); GL= 10 (Low); Net carbs= 19.7 g

Fuji Apples ☛ Serving size= 1 cup, sliced, 109 (g); GI= 36 (Low); GL= 5.1 (Low); Net carbs= 14.3 g

Gala Apples ☛ Serving size= 1 cup, sliced, 109 (g); GI= 39 (Low); GL= 4.8 (Low); Net carbs= 12.4 g

Golden Delicious Apples ☛ Serving size= 1 cup, sliced, 109 (g); GI= 39 (Low); GL= 4.8 (Low); Net carbs= 12.2 g

Gooseberries ☛ Serving size= 1 cup, 150 (g); GI= 21 (Low); GL= 1.9 (Low); Net carbs= 8.8 g

Granny Smith Apples ☛ Serving size= 1 cup, sliced, 109 (g); GI= 36 (Low); GL= 4.2 (Low); Net carbs= 11.8 g

Grapefruit ☛ Serving size= 1 cup sections, with juice, 230 (g); GI= 25 (Low); GL= 4 (Low); Net carbs= 16.1 g

Grapefruit And Orange Sections Cooked Canned Or Frozen—unsweetened Water Pack ☛ Serving size= 1 cup, 244 (g); GI= 75 (High); GL= 10 (Low); Net carbs= 13.4 g

Grapes ☛ Serving size= 1 cup, 92 (g); GI= 53 (Low); GL= 7.9 (Low); Net carbs= 15 g

Green Olives Marinated ☛ Serving size= 1 olive, 2.7 (g); GI= 17 (Low); GL= 0 (Low); Net carbs= 0 g

Groundcherries ☛ Serving size= 1 cup, 140 (g); GI= 35 (Low); GL= 5.5 (Low); Net carbs= 15.7 g

Guavas ☛ Serving size= 1 cup, 165 (g); GI= 24 (Low); GL= 3.5 (Low); Net carbs= 14.7 g

Honeydew Melon ☛ Serving size= 1 cup, diced (approx 20 pieces per cup), 170 (g); GI= 62 (Medium); GL= 8.7 (Low); Net carbs= 14.1 g

Java Plum ☛ Serving size= 1 cup, 135 (g); GI= 25 (Low); GL= 5.3 (Low); Net carbs= 21 g

Kumquats ☛ Serving size= 1 fruit without refuse, 19 (g); GI= 0 (Low); GL= 0 (Low); Net carbs= 1.8 g

Lemon Juice—From Concentrate Bottled ☛ Serving size= 1 tbsp, 15 (g); GI= 55 (Medium); GL= 0.4 (Low); Net carbs= 0.8 g

Lemon Juice—From Concentrate Bottled Real Lemon ☛ Serving size= 1 tbsp, 15 (g); GI= 55 (Medium); GL= 0.4 (Low); Net carbs= 0.7 g

Lemon Juice—From Concentrate Canned Or Bottled ☛ Serving size= 1 tbsp, 15 (g); GI= 55 (Medium); GL= 0.4 (Low); Net carbs= 0.7 g

Lemon Juice—Raw ☛ Serving size= 1 cup, 244 (g); GI= 51 (Low); GL= 8.2 (Low); Net carbs= 16.1 g

Lemon Peel Raw ☛ Serving size= 1 tbsp, 6 (g); GI= 28 (Low); GL= 0.1 (Low); Net carbs= 0.3 g

Lime Juice ☛ Serving size= 1 cup, 242 (g); GI= 51 (Low); GL= 9.9 (Low); Net carbs= 19.4 g

Lime Juice—Canned Or Bottled—unsweetened ☛ Serving size= 1 cup, 246 (g); GI= 51 (Low); GL= 7.9 (Low); Net carbs= 15.5 g

Limes ☛ Serving size= 1 fruit (2 inch dia), 67 (g); GI= 25 (Low); GL= 1.3 (Low); Net carbs= 5.2 g

Lychee Cooked Or Canned In Sugar Or Syrup ☛ Serving size= 1 lychee with liquid, 21 (g); GI= 74 (High); GL= 3.6 (Low); Net carbs= 4.9 g

Mango Pickled ☛ Serving size= 1 slice, 28 (g); GI= 51 (Low); GL= 4.5 (Low); Net carbs= 8.9 g

Maraschino Cherries (Canned) ☛ Serving size= 1 cherry (nlea serving), 5 (g); GI= 85 (High); GL= 1.6 (Low); Net carbs= 1.9 g

Medjool Dates ☛ Serving size= 1 date, pitted, 24 (g); GI= 44 (Low); GL= 7.2 (Low); Net carbs= 16.4 g

Melon Balls ☛ Serving size= 1 cup, unthawed, 173 (g); GI= 62 (Medium); GL= 7.8 (Low); Net carbs= 12.5 g

Mulberries ☛ Serving size= 1 cup, 140 (g); GI= (); GL= 0 (Low); Net carbs= 11.3 g

Mushrooms Pickled ☛ Serving size= 1 cup, 156 (g); GI= (); GL= 0 (Low); Net carbs= 3.1 g

Nance—Canned Syrup Drained ☛ Serving size= 3 fruit without pits, 11.1 (g); GI= 85 (High); GL= 1.5 (Low); Net carbs= 1.8 g

Navel Oranges ☛ Serving size= 1 cup sections, without membranes, 165 (g); GI= 43 (Low); GL= 7.3 (Low); Net carbs= 17.1 g

Nectarines ☛ Serving size= 1 cup slices, 143 (g); GI= 35 (Low); GL= 4.4 (Low); Net carbs= 12.7 g

Olives ☛ Serving size= 1 tbsp, 8.4 (g); GI= 15 (Low); GL= 0.1 (Low); Net carbs= 0.4 g

Olives Black ☛ Serving size= 1 slice, 1 (g); GI= 15 (Low); GL= 0 (Low); Net carbs= 0 g

Olives Green Stuffed ☛ Serving size= 1 cup, 147 (g); GI= 15 (Low); GL= 0.2 (Low); Net carbs= 1.4 g

Oranges ☛ Serving size= 1 cup, sections, 180 (g); GI= 45 (Low); GL= 7.6 (Low); Net carbs= 16.8 g

Oranges Raw With Peel ☛ Serving size= 1 cup, 170 (g); GI= 45 (Low); GL= 8.4 (Low); Net carbs= 18.7 g

Papaya ☛ Serving size= 1 cup 1 inch pieces, 145 (g); GI= 60 (Medium); GL= 7.9 (Low); Net carbs= 13.2 g

Passion Fruit (Granadilla) ☛ Serving size= 1 cup, 236 (g); GI= 30 (Low); GL= 9.2 (Low); Net carbs= 30.6 g

Peach Pickled ☛ Serving size= 1 fruit, 88 (g); GI= 40 (Low); GL= 9.9 (Low); Net carbs= 24.8 g

Peaches—Canned Water Pack Solids And Liquids ☛ Serving size= 1 cup, halves or slices, 244 (g); GI= 81 (High); GL= 9.5 (Low); Net carbs= 11.7 g

Pears ☛ Serving size= 1 cup, slices, 140 (g); GI= 33 (Low); GL= 5.6 (Low); Net carbs= 17 g

Persimmons Native Raw ☛ Serving size= 1 fruit without refuse, 25 (g); GI= 61 (Medium); GL= 5.1 (Low); Net carbs= 8.4 g

Plum Pickled ☛ Serving size= 1 plum, 28 (g); GI= 24 (Low); GL= 2 (Low); Net carbs= 8.3 g

Plums ☛ Serving size= 1 cup, sliced, 165 (g); GI= 24 (Low); GL= 4 (Low); Net carbs= 16.5 g

Pomegranates ☛ Serving size= 1/2 cup arils (seed/juice sacs), 87 (g); GI= 53 (Low); GL= 6.8 (Low); Net carbs= 12.8 g

Prune Dried Cooked Without Sugar ☛ Serving size= 1 prune, 10 (g); GI= 39 (Low); GL= 1.3 (Low); Net carbs= 3.3 g

Prune Puree ☛ Serving size= 2 tbsp, 36 (g); GI= 43 (Low); GL= 9.6 (Low); Net carbs= 22.2 g

Pummelo ☛ Serving size= 1 cup, sections, 190 (g); GI= 22 (Low); GL= 3.6 (Low); Net carbs= 16.4 g

Quinces ☛ Serving size= 1 fruit without refuse, 92 (g); GI= 35 (Low); GL= 4.3 (Low); Net carbs= 12.3 g

Raspberries ☛ Serving size= 1 cup, 123 (g); GI= 78 (High); GL= 5.2 (Low); Net carbs= 6.7 g

Raspberries Cooked Or Canned—unsweetened Water Pack ☛ Serving size= 1 cup, 243 (g); GI= 77 (High); GL= 6.7 (Low); Net carbs= 8.7 g

Raspberries Frozen—unsweetened ☛ Serving size= 1 cup, 250 (g); GI= 32 (Low); GL= 4.4 (Low); Net carbs= 13.6 g

Red And White Currants ☛ Serving size= 1 cup, 112 (g); GI= 25 (Low); GL= 2.7 (Low); Net carbs= 10.6 g

Red Delicious Apples ☛ Serving size= 1 cup, sliced, 109 (g); GI= 39 (Low); GL= 5 (Low); Net carbs= 12.8 g

Rhubarb ☛ Serving size= 1 cup, diced, 122 (g); GI= 15 (Low); GL= 0.5 (Low); Net carbs= 3.3 g

Rhubarb Cooked Or Canned—unsweetened ☛ Serving size= 1 cup, 240 (g); GI= 17 (Low); GL= 1.1 (Low); Net carbs= 6.6 g

Rhubarb Frozen Uncooked ☛ Serving size= 1 cup, diced, 137 (g); GI= 15 (Low); GL= 0.7 (Low); Net carbs= 4.5 g

Sour Red Cherries ☛ Serving size= 1 cup, without pits, 155 (g); GI= 22 (Low); GL= 3.6 (Low); Net carbs= 16.4 g

Sour Red Cherries (Frozen) ☛ Serving size= 1 cup, unthawed, 155 (g); GI= 22 (Low); GL= 3.2 (Low); Net carbs= 14.6 g

Starfruit (Carambola) ☛ Serving size= 1 cup, cubes, 132 (g); GI= 45 (Low); GL= 2.3 (Low); Net carbs= 5.2 g

Strawberries ☛ Serving size= 1 cup, halves, 152 (g); GI= 41 (Low); GL= 3.5 (Low); Net carbs= 8.6 g

Strawberries Cooked Or Canned—unsweetened Water Pack ☛ Serving size= 1 cup, 242 (g); GI= 75 (High); GL= 7 (Low); Net carbs= 9.3 g

Tangerines (Mandarin Oranges)—Canned Juice—Pack Drained ☛ Serving size= 1 cup, 189 (g); GI= 59 (Medium); GL= 9.2 (Low); Net carbs= 15.5 g

Watermelon ☛ Serving size= 1 cup, balls, 154 (g); GI= 72 (High); GL= 7.9 (Low); Net carbs= 11 g

34
GRAINS AND PASTA

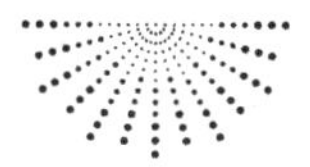

Barley—Fat Added In Cooking ☛ Serving size= 1 cup, cooked (170 g); GI= 25 (Low); GL= 10 (Low); Net carb= 40 g

Bulgur (cooked with added fat) ☛ Serving size= 1 cup, cooked (140 g); GI= 47 (Low); GL= 8.6 (Low); Net carb= 18.4 g

Bulgur (cooked without added fat) ☛ Serving size= 1 cup, cooked (140 g); GI= 47 (Low); GL= 9.2 (Low); Net carb= 19.6 g

Corn Bran Crude ☛ Serving size= 1 cup (76 g); GI= 75 (High); GL= 3.8 (Low); Net carb= 5 g

Flour—Corn, Whole-Grain Blue (Harina De Maiz Morado) ☛ Serving size= 1 tbsp (6.9 g); GI= 55 (Medium); GL= 2.5 (Low); Net carb= 4.6 g

Hominy Canned Yellow ☛ Serving size= 1 cup (160 g); GI= 40 (Low); GL= 7.5 (Low); Net carb= 18.8 g

Noodles—Chinese Chow Mein ☛ Serving size= 1/2 cup dry (28 g); GI= 35 (Low); GL= 5.6 (Low); Net carb= 15.9 g

Noodles—Japanese Soba (Buckwheat) ☛ Serving size= 1 cup (114 g); GI= 41 (Low); GL= 10 (Low); Net carb= 24.4 g

Noodles—Rice (Cooked) ☛ Serving size= 2 oz (57 g); GI= 56 (Medium); GL= 7.3 (Low); Net carb= 13.1 g

Pasta—Fresh-Refrigerated Spinach Cooked ☛ Serving size= 2 oz (57 g); GI= 58 (Medium); GL= 8.3 (Low); Net carb= 14.3 g

Pasta—Homemade Made With Egg Cooked ☛ Serving size= 2 oz (57 g); GI= 66 (Medium); GL= 8.9 (Low); Net carb= 13.4 g

Pasta—Homemade Made Without Egg Cooked ☛ Serving size= 2 oz (57 g); GI= 66 (Medium); GL= 9.5 (Low); Net carb= 14.3 g

Rice Brown—Parboiled Dry Uncle Bens ☛ Serving size= 1/4 cup (48 g); GI= 38 (Low); GL= 3.4 (Low); Net carb= 9 g

Spaghetti—Spinach Cooked ☛ Serving size= 2 oz (57 g); GI= 33 (Low); GL= 4.9 (Low); Net carb= 14.9 g

White Rice (average for grain length) ☛ Serving size= 1/4 cup (48 g); GI= 69 (Medium); GL= 9.2 (Low); Net carb= 13.3 g

35

HERBS AND SPICES

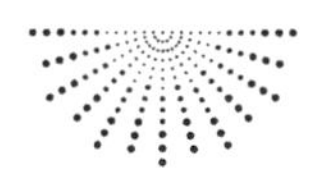

Allspice ☛ Serving size= 1 tsp (2.1 g) ; GI= 15 (Low); GL= 0.3 (Low)

Anise seeds ☛ Serving size= 1 tsp (2.1 g) ; GI= 0.0 (Low); GL= 0.3 (Low)

Asian chives ☛ Serving size= 1 tbsp (3 g); GI= 15 (Low); GL= 0.3 (Low)

Basil ☛ Serving size= 1 tsp (0.7 g); GI= 70 (High); GL= 0 (Low)

Bay leaves ☛ Serving size= 1 tbsp, crumbled (1.8 g); GI= 23 (Low); GL= 0.1 (Low)

Black cumin ☛ Serving size= 1 tsp (2.4 g) ; GI= 0.0 (Low); GL= 0.3 (Low)

Black pepper ☛ Serving size= 1 tsp (2.4 g) ; GI= 44 (Low); GL= 0.3 (Low)

capers ☛ Serving size= 1 tbsp (8.6 g); GI= 20 (Low); GL= 1.4 (Low)

Caraway ☛ Serving size= 1 tbsp (6.7 g); GI= 5 (Low); GL= 1.1 (Low)

Cardamom ☛ Serving size= 1 tbsp (5.8 g); GI= 82 (High); GL= 1 (Low)

Cayenne pepper

☛ Serving size= 1 tsp (2.4 g) ; GI= 32 (Low); GL= 0.4 (Low)

Celery seed ☛ Serving size= 1 tbsp (5.8 g); GI= 32 (Low); GL= 0.9 (Low)

Chiles ☛ Serving size= 1 tbsp (8 g); GI= 42 (Low); GL= 1.3 (Low)

chilli ☛ Serving size= 1 tbsp (8 g); GI= 15 (Low); GL= 1.3 (Low)

Chives ☛ Serving size= 1 tbsp (2.8 g); GI= 15 (Low); GL= 0.3 (Low)

Cilantro

☛ Serving size= 1 cup (16 g); GI= 32 (Low); GL= 0 (Low)

Cinnamon ☛ Serving size= 1 tbsp (7.9 g) ; GI= 70 (High); GL= 2.1 (Low)

Cloves ☛ Serving size= 1 tbsp (6.6 g); GI= 87 (High); GL= 3.5 (Low)

Coriander seed ☛ Serving size= 1 tbsp (5 g) ; GI= 33 (Low); GL= 1 (Low)

Cumin ☛ Serving size= 1 tbsp (6 g); GI= 0.0 (Low); GL= 0 (Low)

Curry Leaves ☛ Serving size= 5 leaves (2g); GI= 5 (Low); GL= 0.1 (Low)

Curry powder ☛ Serving size= 1 tbsp (6 g); GI= 5 (Low); GL= 0.4 (Low)

Dill seed ☛ Serving size= 1 tsp (2.4 g) ; GI= 15 (Low); GL= 0.3 (Low)

Fennel seeds ☛ Serving size= 1 tbsp (5.8 g); GI= 16 (Low); GL= 0.3 (Low)

Fenugreek ☛ Serving size= 1 tbsp (11.1 g) ; GI= 25 (Low); GL= 0.6 (Low)

Fenugreek Leaves ☛ Serving size= 1 cup (85 g); GI= 25 (Low); GL= 0.6 (Low)

Five Spice Powder ☛ Serving size= 1 tsp (2.1 g) ; GI= 15 (Low); GL= 0.4 (Low)

Garlic chives ☛ Serving size= 2 clove (6 g); GI= 15 (Low); GL= 1 (Low)

Ginger ☛ Serving size= 1 tsp (2.1 g) ; GI= 72 (High); GL= 0.3 (Low)

Lemon Balm ☛ Serving size= 1 tsp (2.1 g) ; GI= 15 (Low); GL= 0.3 (Low)

Lemongrass ☛ Serving size= 1 cup (67 g); GI= 45 (Low); GL= 7.4 (Low)

Lime Leaves ☛ Serving size= 5 leaves (2 g); GI= 32 (Low); GL= 0.4 (Low)

Mint ☛ Serving size= 1 tbsp (3.1 g) ; GI= 10 (Low); GL= 0.2 (Low)

Mustard Seed ☛ Serving size= 1 tsp (2 g) ; GI= 32 (Low); GL= 0.2 (Low)

Nutmeg ☛ Serving size= 1 tsp (2.4 g) ; GI= 46 (Low); GL= 0.3 (Low)

Oregano ☛ Serving size= 1 tbsp (3 g); GI= 5 (Low); GL= 0.3 (Low)

Paprika ☛ Serving size= 1 tsp (2 g) ; GI= 15 (Low); GL= 0.3 (Low)

Parsley

☛ Serving size= 1 tbsp (3 g); GI= 32 (Low); GL= 0.3 (Low)

Poppy seeds ☛ Serving size= 1 tbsp (8.8 g); GI= 5 (Low); GL= 0.1 (Low)

Rosemary ☛ Serving size= 1 tbsp (3.3 g); GI= 70 (High); GL= 1.1 (Low)

Saffron ☛ Serving size= 1 tsp (0.7 g); GI= 70 (High); GL= 0.2 (Low)

Sage ☛ Serving size= 1 tsp (0.7 g); GI= 15 (Low); GL= 0.2 (Low)

Savory ☛ Serving size= 1 tbsp (4.4 g); GI= 16 (Low); GL= 0.2 (Low)

Sesame seeds ☛ Serving size= 1 tbsp (10 g); GI= 31 (Low); GL= 0.1 (Low)

Sumac ☛ Serving size= 1 tsp (2.7 g) ; GI= 43 (Low); GL= 0.2 (Low)

Summer Savoy ☛ Serving size= 1 tsp (2.7 g) ; GI= 21 (Low); GL= 0.2 (Low)

Tarragon ☛ Serving size= 1 tbsp (1.8g); GI= 15 (Low); GL= 0.1 (Low)

Thyme ☛ Serving size= 1 tbsp, leaves (2.7 g); GI= 51 (Low); GL= 0.1 (Low)

Turmeric ☛ Serving size= 1 tbsp (6.8 g); GI= 15 (Low); GL= 0.5 (Low)

Vanilla ☛ Serving size= 1 tbsp (4.4 g); GI= 16 (Low); GL= 0.5 (Low)

Wasabi powder ☛ Serving size= 1 tsp (2.8 g); GI= 31 (Low); GL= 0.3 (Low)

Watercress ☛ Serving size= 1 cup, chopped (34 g); GI= 32 (Low); GL= 0.1 (Low)

Wild garlic ☛ Serving size= 1 oz (28 g); GI= 11 (Low); GL= 2 (Low)

36
VEGETABLES

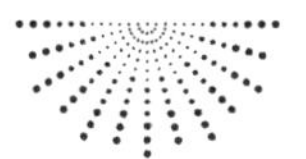

Alfalfa sprouts, raw ☛ GI= 32 (Low); Serving size= 1 cup (33 g); GL= 0.3 (Low); Net carb= 0.2 g

Algae, dried ☛ GI= 32 (Low); Serving size= 1 serv (7 g); GL= 1 (Low); Net carb= 3 g

Artichoke— globe (French), cooked, from fresh, with fat ☛ GI= 32 (Low); Serving size= 1 medium globe (103 g); GL= 1.4 (Low); Net carb= 4.5 g

Artichoke— globe (French), cooked, from fresh, without fat ☛ GI= 32 (Low); Serving size= 1 medium globe (103 g); GL= 1.4 (Low); Net carb= 4.5 g

Artichoke— Jerusalem, raw ☛ GI= 32 (Low); Serving size= 1 whole artichoke (173 g); GL= 2.4 (Low); Net carb= 7.6 g

Artichoke— salad in oil ☛ GI= 32 (Low); Serving size= 1 medium globe (103 g); GL= 1.4 (Low); Net carb= 4.5 g

Asparagus— cooked, from canned, with fat ☛ GI= 32 (Low); Serving size= 8 spears (134 g); GL= 0.6 (Low); Net carb= 1.8 g

Asparagus— cooked, from canned, without fat ☛ GI= 32 (Low); Serving size= 8 spears (134 g); GL= 0.6 (Low); Net carb= 1.8 g

Asparagus— cooked, from fresh, with fat ☛ GI= 32 (Low); Serving size= 8 spears (134 g); GL= 0.6 (Low); Net carb= 1.8 g

Asparagus— cooked, from fresh, without fat ☛ GI= 32 (Low); Serving size= 8 spears (134 g); GL= 0.6 (Low); Net carb= 1.8 g

Asparagus— cooked—From Frozen, with fat ☛ GI= 32 (Low); Serving size= 8 spears (134 g); GL= 0.6 (Low); Net carb= 1.8 g

Asparagus— cooked—From Frozen, without fat ☛ GI= 32 (Low); Serving size= 8 spears (134 g); GL= 0.6 (Low); Net carb= 1.8 g

Asparagus— from canned, creamed or with cheese sauce ☛ GI= 28 (Low); Serving size= 8 spears (134 g); GL= 0.5 (Low); Net carb= 1.8 g

Asparagus— from fresh, creamed or with cheese sauce ☛ GI= 29 (Low); Serving size= 8 spears (134 g); GL= 0.5 (Low); Net carb= 1.8 g

Asparagus— raw ☛ GI= 32 (Low); Serving size= 8 spears (134 g); GL= 0.6 (Low); Net carb= 1.8 g

Bamboo shoots—cooked, with fat ☛ GI= 32 (Low); Serving size= 1 cup (155 grams); GL= 0.4 (Low); Net carb= 6 g

Bamboo shoots—cooked, without fat ☛ GI= 32 (Low); Serving size= 1 cup (155 grams); GL= 0.6 (Low); Net carb= 6 g

Bean sprouts— cooked, from canned, with fat ☛ GI= 32 (Low); Serving size= 1 cup, canned (129 g); GL= 1.7 (Low); Net carb= 5.4 g

Bean sprouts— cooked, from canned, without fat ☛ GI= 32 (Low); Serving size= 1 cup, canned (129 g); GL= 1.7 (Low); Net carb= 5.4 g

Bean sprouts— cooked, from fresh, with fat ☛ GI= 32 (Low); Serving size= 1 cup (129 g); GL= 1.7 (Low); Net carb= 5.4 g

Bean sprouts— cooked, from fresh, without fat ☛ GI= 32 (Low); Serving size= 1 cup (129 g); GL= 1.7 (Low); Net carb= 5.4 g

Bean sprouts— raw (soybean or mung) ☛ GI= 32 (Low); Serving size= 1 cup (129 g); GL= 1.7 (Low); Net carb= 5.4 g

Beet greens—raw ☛ GI= 32 (Low); Serving size= 1 cup (124 g); GL= 1.7 (Low); Net carb= 5.4 g

Beets— cooked, from canned, with fat ☛ GI= 64 (Medium); Serving size= 1 cup, canned (157 g); GL= 8.2 (Low); Net carb= 12.8 g

Beets— cooked, from canned, without fat ☛ GI= 64 (Medium); Serving size= 1 cup, canned (157 g); GL= 8.2 (Low); Net carb= 12.8 g

Beets— cooked, from fresh, without fat ☛ GI= 64 (Medium); Serving size= 1 cup, diced (157 g); GL= 8.2 (Low); Net carb= 12.8 g

Beets— pickled ☛ GI= 66 (Medium); Serving size= 1 cup, diced (157 g); GL= 8.4 (Low); Net carb= 12.8 g

Beets— raw ☛ GI= 64 (Medium); Serving size= 1 cup, diced (157 g); GL= 8.2 (Low); Net carb= 12.8 g

Beets—with Harvard sauce ☛ GI= 66 (Medium); Serving size= 1 cup, diced (157 g); GL= 8.5 (Low); Net carb= 12.8 g

Bitter melon—cooked, without fat ☛ GI= 32 (Low); Serving size= 1 cup (93 g); GL= 0.7 (Low); Net carb= 2.3 g

Broccoflower—Cooked—Made With Butter ☛ GI= 32 (Low); Serving size= 1 cup (87 g); GL= 0.8 (Low); Net carb= 2.6 g

Broccoflower—Cooked—Made With Oil ☛ GI= 32 (Low); Serving size= 1 cup (87 g); GL= 0.8 (Low); Net carb= 2.6 g

Broccoflower—cooked, without fat ☛ GI= 32 (Low); Serving size= 1 cup (87 g); GL= 0.8 (Low); Net carb= 2.6 g

Broccoli—cooked, from fresh, without fat ☛ GI= 32 (Low); Serving size= 1 medium stalk (148 g); GL= 1.9 (Low); Net carb= 5.9 g

Broccoli—cooked—From Frozen, without fat ☛ GI= 32 (Low); Serving size= 1 medium stalk (148 g); GL= 1.9 (Low); Net carb= 5.9 g

Broccoli—raw ☛ GI= 32 (Low); Serving size= 1 medium stalk (148 g); GL= 1.9 (Low); Net carb= 5.9 g

Brussels sprouts—cooked, from fresh, without fat ☛ GI= 32 (Low); Serving size= 1 cup (160 g); GL= 2.3 (Low); Net carb= 7.2 g

Brussels sprouts—cooked—From Frozen, without fat ☛ GI= 32 (Low); Serving size= 1 cup (160 g); GL= 2.3 (Low); Net carb= 7.2 g

Brussels sprouts—raw ☛ GI= 32 (Low); Serving size= 1 cup (160 g); GL= 2.3 (Low); Net carb= 7.2 g

Cabbage—Chinese, cooked, with fat ☛ GI= 32 (Low); Serving size= 1 cup, shredded (170 g); GL= 0.4 (Low); Net carb= 1.4 g

Cabbage—Chinese, cooked, without fat ☛ GI= 32 (Low); Serving size= 1 cup, shredded (170 g); GL= 0.4 (Low); Net carb= 1.4 g

Cabbage—Chinese, raw ☛ GI= 32 (Low); Serving size= 1 cup, shredded (170 g); GL= 0.4 (Low); Net carb= 1.4 g

Cabbage—fresh, pickled, Japanese style ☛ GI= 32 (Low); Serving size= 1 cup (150 g); GL= 1.2 (Low); Net carb= 3.9 g

Cabbage—green, cooked, with fat ☛ GI= 32 (Low); Serving size= 1 cup (150 g); GL= 1.7 (Low); Net carb= 5.3 g

Cabbage—green, cooked, without fat ☛ GI= 32 (Low); Serving size= 1 cup (150 g); GL= 1.7 (Low); Net carb= 5.3 g

Cabbage—green, raw ☛ GI= 32 (Low); Serving size= 1 cup (150 g); GL= 1.7 (Low); Net carb= 5.3 g

Cabbage—Kim Chee style ☛ GI= 32 (Low); Serving size= 1 cup (150 g); GL= 1.7 (Low); Net carb= 5.3 g

Cabbage—red, cooked, with fat ☛ GI= 32 (Low); Serving size= 1 cup (150 g); GL= 1.7 (Low); Net carb= 5.3 g

Cabbage—red, cooked, without fat ☛ GI= 32 (Low); Serving size= 1 cup (150 g); GL= 1.7 (Low); Net carb= 5.3 g

Cabbage—red, pickled ☛ GI= 32 (Low); Serving size= 1 cup (150 g); GL= 1.7 (Low); Net carb= 5.3 g

Cabbage—red, raw ☛ GI= 32 (Low); Serving size= 1 cup (150 g); GL= 1.7 (Low); Net carb= 5.3 g

Cactus—cooked, with fat ☛ GI= 7 (Low); Serving size= 1 cup (150 g); GL= 0.1 (Low); Net carb= 1.9 g

Cactus—cooked, without fat ☛ GI= 7 (Low); Serving size= 1 cup (150 g); GL= 0.1 (Low); Net carb= 1.9 g

Cactus—raw ☛ GI= 7 (Low); Serving size= 1 cup (150 g); GL= 0.1 (Low); Net carb= 1.9 g

Calabaza (Spanish pumpkin), cooked ☛ GI= 75 (High); Serving size= 1 cup, cubes (166 g); GL= 6.2 (Low); Net carb= 8.3 g

Carrots—canned, low sodium, without fat ☛ GI= 47 (Low); Serving size= 1 cup, canned (151 g); GL= 4.3 (Low); Net carb= 9.2 g

Carrots—cooked, from canned, without fat ☛ GI= 47 (Low); Serving size= 1 cup or 1 carrot, 7" long (151 g); GL= 4.3 (Low); Net carb= 9.2 g

Carrots—cooked, from fresh, without fat ☛ GI= 47 (Low); Serving size= 1 cup or 1 carrot, 7" long (151 g); GL= 4.3 (Low); Net carb= 9.2 g

Carrots—cooked—From Frozen, without fat ☛ GI= 47 (Low); Serving size= 1 cup or 1 carrot, 7" long (151 g); GL= 4.3 (Low); Net carb= 9.2 g

Carrots—raw ☛ GI= 47 (Low); Serving size= 1 cup or 1 carrot, 7" long (151 g); GL= 4.8 (Low); Net carb= 10.2 g

Cauliflower—cooked, from fresh, without fat ☛ GI= 32 (Low); Serving size= 1 cup chopped (107 g); GL= 0.6 (Low); Net carb= 1.9 g

Cauliflower—cooked—From Frozen, without fat ☛ GI= 32 (Low); Serving size= 1 cup chopped (107 g); GL= 0.6 (Low); Net carb= 1.9 g

Cauliflower—pickled ☛ GI= 32 (Low); Serving size= 1 cup chopped (107 g); GL= 0.6 (Low); Net carb= 1.9 g

Cauliflower—raw ☛ GI= 32 (Low); Serving size= 1 cup chopped (107 g); GL= 0.6 (Low); Net carb= 1.9 g

Celery juice ☛ GI= 32 (Low); Serving size= 1 cup (240 g); GL= 1.8 (Low); Net carb= 5.5 g

Celery—cooked, with fat ☛ GI= 32 (Low); Serving size= 1 cup, diced (150 g); GL= 1.1 (Low); Net carb= 3.5 g

Celery—cooked, without fat ☛ GI= 32 (Low); Serving size= 1 cup, diced (150 g); GL= 1.1 (Low); Net carb= 3.5 g

Celery—raw ☛ GI= 32 (Low); Serving size= 1 cup, diced (150 g); GL= 1.1 (Low); Net carb= 3.5 g

Chard, cooked, without fat ☛ GI= 32 (Low); Serving size= 1 cup, stalk and leaves (150 grams); GL= 1 (Low); Net carb= 3 g

Christophine—cooked, without fat ☛ GI= 32 (Low); Serving size= 1 cup (165 g); GL= 1.2 (Low); Net carb= 3.8 g

Christophine—cooked, without fat ☛ GI= 32 (Low); Serving size= 1 cup (165 g); GL= 1.2 (Low); Net carb= 3.8 g

Coleslaw, with dressing ☛ GI= 44 (Low); Serving size= 1 cup (120 g); GL= 5.8 (Low); Net carb= 13.2 g

Collards—cooked, from canned, without fat ☛ GI= 32 (Low); Serving size= 1 cup, canned (170 g); GL= 2.3 (Low); Net carb= 7.3 g

Collards—cooked, from fresh, without fat ☛ GI= 32 (Low); Serving size= 1 cup, canned (170 g); GL= 2.3 (Low); Net carb= 7.3 g

Collards, cooked—From Frozen, without fat ☛ GI= 32 (Low); Serving size= 1 cup, canned (170 g); GL= 2.3 (Low); Net carb= 7.3 g

Corn Dried Cooked ☛ GI= 48 (Low); Serving size= 1 oz (28 g); GL= 1.8 (Low); Net carb= 3.8 g

Corn Sweet Yellow—Canned—Drained Solids Rinsed With Tap Water

☛ GI= 52 (Low); Serving size= 1 cup (150 g); GL= 8.8 (Low); Net carb= 17 g

Cucumber salad—made with Cucumber—oil, and vinegar ☛ GI= 32 (Low); Serving size= 1 cup (185 g); GL= 2.3 (Low); Net carb= 7.2 g

Cucumber salad—with creamy dressing ☛ GI= 32 (Low); Serving size= 1 cup (185 g); GL= 2.3 (Low); Net carb= 7.2 g

Cucumber—cooked, with fat ☛ GI= 32 (Low); Serving size= 1 cup (185 g); GL= 2.3 (Low); Net carb= 7.2 g

Cucumber—cooked, without fat ☛ GI= 32 (Low); Serving size= 1 cup (185 g); GL= 2.3 (Low); Net carb= 7.2 g

Cucumber—pickles, dill ☛ GI= 32 (Low); Serving size= 1 cup (185 g); GL= 2.3 (Low); Net carb= 7.2 g

Cucumber—pickles, fresh ☛ GI= 32 (Low); Serving size= 1 cup (185 g); GL= 2.3 (Low); Net carb= 7.2 g

Cucumber—pickles, relish ☛ GI= 32 (Low); Serving size= 1 cup (185 g); GL= 2.3 (Low); Net carb= 7.2 g

Cucumber—raw ☛ GI= 32 (Low); Serving size= 1 cup, pared, chopped (133 g); GL= 1.7 (Low); Net carb= 5.2 g

Cucumber,pickles, sour ☛ GI= 32 (Low); Serving size= 1 medium, 3 3/4" long (65g); GL= 0.2 (Low); Net carb= 0.8 g

Cucumber,pickles, sweet ☛ GI= 32 (Low); Serving size= 1 medium, 3 3/4" long (65g); GL= 0.2 (Low); Net carb= 0.8 g

Dandelion greens—cooked, without fat ☛ GI= 32 (Low); Serving size= 1 cup, chopped (110 grams); GL= 1.2 (Low); Net carb= 3.9 g

Dandelion greens—raw ☛ GI= 32 (Low); Serving size= 1 cup (55 grams); GL= 0.6 (Low); Net carb= 1.9 g

Eggplant—cooked, tomato sauce, without fat ☛ GI= 35 (Low); Serving size= 1 cup (155 g); GL= 3.5 (Low); Net carb= 10.1 g

Eggplant—cooked, with fat ☛ GI= 32 (Low); Serving size= 1 cup (155 g); GL= 2.8 (Low); Net carb= 8.7 g

Eggplant—cooked, without fat ☛ GI= 32 (Low); Serving size= 1 cup (155 g); GL= 2.8 (Low); Net carb= 8.7 g

Eggplant—pickled ☛ GI= 32 (Low); Serving size= 1 cup (155 g); GL= 2.8 (Low); Net carb= 8.7 g

Endive—raw ☛ GI= 32 (Low); Serving size= 1 cup, chopped (50 g); GL= 0.1 (Low); Net carb= 0.3 g

Fennel ☛ GI= 16 (Low); Serving size= 1 cup, sliced (87 g); GL= 0.6 (Low); Net carb= 3.7 g

Fennel Bulb—Cooked—(cooked with fat) (average) ☛ GI= 16 (Low); Serving size= 1 fennel bulb (218 g); GL= 2.3 (Low); Net carb= 14.1 g

Fennel Bulb—Cooked—(cooked without fat) ☛ GI= 16 (Low); Serving size= 1 fennel bulb (218 g); GL= 2.3 (Low); Net carb= 14.4 g

Fennel Bulb—Cooked—Made With Butter ☛ GI= 16 (Low); Serving size= 1 fennel bulb (218 g); GL= 2.3 (Low); Net carb= 14.1 g

Fennel Bulb—Cooked—Made With Oil ☛ GI= 16 (Low); Serving size= 1 fennel bulb (218 g); GL= 2.3 (Low); Net carb= 14.1 g

Escarole—cooked, without fat ☛ GI= 32 (Low); Serving size= 1 cup (135 g); GL= 0.1 (Low); Net carb= 0.4 g

Greens—cooked, from canned, without fat ☛ GI= 32 (Low); Serving size= 1 cup, canned (170 g); GL= 1 (Low); Net carb= 3.2 g

Greens—cooked, from fresh, without fat ☛ GI= 32 (Low); Serving size= 1 cup (175 g); GL= 1 (Low); Net carb= 3.2 g

Jicama—raw ☛ GI= 22 (Low); Serving size= 1 cup (130 g); GL= 1.5 (Low); Net carb= 6.6 g

Kale ☛ GI= 32 (Low); Serving size= 1 cup 1 inch pieces (16 g); GL= 0 (Low); Net carb= 0.1 g

Kale—Cooked From Canned—(cooked with fat) (average) ☛ GI= 32 (Low); Serving size= 1 cup, canned (168 g); GL= 1.9 (Low); Net carb= 5.9 g

Kale—Cooked From Canned—(cooked without fat) ☛ GI= 32 (Low); Serving size= 1 cup, canned (163 g); GL= 1.9 (Low); Net carb= 5.9 g

Kale—Cooked From Canned—Made With Butter ☛ GI= 32 (Low); Serving size= 1 cup, canned (168 g); GL= 1.9 (Low); Net carb= 5.9 g

Kale—Cooked From Canned—Made With Oil ☛ GI= 32 (Low); Serving size= 1 cup, canned (168 g); GL= 1.9 (Low); Net carb= 5.9 g

Kale—Cooked From Fresh—(cooked with fat) (average) ☛ GI= 32 (Low); Serving size= 1 cup, fresh (135 g); GL= 1.5 (Low); Net carb= 4.7 g

Kale—Cooked From Fresh—(cooked without fat) ☛ GI= 32 (Low); Serving size= 1 cup, fresh (130 g); GL= 1.5 (Low); Net carb= 4.7 g

Kale—Cooked From Fresh—Made With Butter ☛ GI= 32 (Low); Serving size= 1 cup, fresh (135 g); GL= 1.5 (Low); Net carb= 4.7 g

Kale—Cooked From Fresh—Made With Oil ☛ GI= 32 (Low); Serving size= 1 cup, fresh (135 g); GL= 1.5 (Low); Net carb= 4.7 g

Kale—Cooked From Frozen—(cooked with fat) (average) ☛ GI= 32 (Low); Serving size= 1 cup, frozen (135 g); GL= 1.3 (Low); Net carb= 4.2 g

Kale—Cooked From Frozen—(cooked without fat) ☛ GI= 32 (Low); Serving size= 1 cup, frozen (130 g); GL= 1.3 (Low); Net carb= 4.1 g

Kale—Cooked From Frozen—Made With Butter ☛ GI= 32 (Low); Serving size= 1 cup, frozen (135 g); GL= 1.3 (Low); Net carb= 4.2 g

Kale—Cooked From Frozen—Made With Oil ☛ GI= 32 (Low); Serving size= 1 cup, frozen (135 g); GL= 1.3 (Low); Net carb= 4.2 g

Kale—Cooked NS Form (cooked with fat) (average) ☛ GI= 32 (Low); Serving size= 1 cup (135 g); GL= 1.5 (Low); Net carb= 4.7 g

Kale—Cooked NS Form (cooked without fat) ☛ GI= 32 (Low); Serving size= 1 cup (135 g); GL= 1.6 (Low); Net carb= 4.8 g

Kohlrabi ☛ GI= 21 (Low); Serving size= 1 cup (135 g); GL= 0.7 (Low); Net carb= 3.5 g

Kohlrabi—Cooked—(cooked with fat) ☛ GI= 21 (Low); Serving size= 1 cup (170 g); GL= 1.9 (Low); Net carb= 9.1 g

Kohlrabi—Cooked—(cooked without fat) ☛ GI= 21 (Low); Serving size= 1 cup (165 g); GL= 1.9 (Low); Net carb= 9.2 g

Kohlrabi Creamed ☛ GI= 21 (Low); Serving size= 1 cup (187 g); GL= 2.8 (Low); Net carb= 13.2 g

Kale—Frozen—Unprepared ☛ GI= 32 (Low); Serving size= 1/ 3 package (10 oz) (94 g); GL= 0.9 (Low); Net carb= 2.7 g

Leeks ☛ GI= 32 (Low); Serving size= 1 cup slices (165 g); GL= 6.5 (Low); Net carb= 20.4 g

Lettuce—arugula, raw ☛ GI= 32 (Low); Serving size= 1/6 medium head (89 g); GL= 0.7 (Low); Net carb= 2.3 g

Lettuce—Boston, raw ☛ GI= 32 (Low); Serving size= 1/6 medium head (89 g); GL= 0.7 (Low); Net carb= 2.3 g

Lettuce—cooked, without fat ☛ GI= 32 (Low); Serving size= 1/6 medium head (89 g); GL= 0.7 (Low); Net carb= 2.3 g

Lettuce—raw ☛ GI= 32 (Low); Serving size= 1/6 medium head (89 g); GL= 0.7 (Low); Net carb= 2.3 g

Lotus Root ☛ GI= 34 (Low); Serving size= 10 slices (2 1/2 inch dia) (81 g); GL= 3.4 (Low); Net carb= 10 g

Lotus Root—Cooked—(cooked with fat) ☛ GI= 34 (Low); Serving size= 1 cup (125 g); GL= 5 (Low); Net carb= 14.8 g

Lotus Root—Cooked—(cooked without fat) ☛ GI= 34 (Low); Serving size= 1 cup (120 g); GL= 5.2 (Low); Net carb= 15.3 g

Mushrooms—Cooked—From Canned—(cooked without fat) ☛ GI= 22 (Low); Serving size= 5 medium (89 g); GL= 0.5 (Low); Net carb= 2.4 g

Mushrooms—Cooked—From Canned—Made With Butter ☛ GI= 22 (Low); Serving size= 5 medium (89 g); GL= 0.5 (Low); Net carb= 2.3 g

Mushrooms—Cooked—From Canned—Made With Oil ☛ GI= 22 (Low); Serving size= 5 medium (89 g); GL= 0.5 (Low); Net carb= 2.3 g

Mushrooms—Cooked—From Fresh—(cooked without fat) ☛ GI= 22 (Low); Serving size= 5 medium (89 g); GL= 0.6 (Low); Net carb= 2.7 g

Mushrooms—Cooked—From Fresh—Made With Butter ☛ GI= 22 (Low); Serving size= 5 medium (89 g); GL= 0.6 (Low); Net carb= 2.7 g

Mushrooms—Cooked—From Fresh—Made With Oil ☛ GI= 22 (Low); Serving size= 5 medium (89 g); GL= 0.6 (Low); Net carb= 2.7 g

Mushrooms—Cooked—From Frozen—(cooked without fat) ☛ GI= 22 (Low); Serving size= 5 medium (89 g); GL= 0.6 (Low); Net carb= 2.7 g

Mushrooms—Cooked—From Frozen—Made With Butter ☛ GI= 22 (Low); Serving size= 5 medium (89 g); GL= 0.6 (Low); Net carb= 2.7 g

Mushrooms—Cooked—From Frozen—Made With Oil ☛ GI= 22 (Low); Serving size= 5 medium (89 g); GL= 0.6 (Low); Net carb= 2.7 g

Mushrooms From Canned—Creamed ☛ GI= 22 (Low); Serving size= 1 cup (217 g); GL= 2.6 (Low); Net carb= 11.9 g

Mushrooms From Fresh—Creamed ☛ GI= 22 (Low); Serving size= 1 cup (217 g); GL= 2.7 (Low); Net carb= 12.4 g

Mushrooms From Frozen—Creamed ☛ GI= 22 (Low); Serving size= 1 cup (217 g); GL= 2.7 (Low); Net carb= 12.4 g

Mushrooms Portobellos Grilled ☛ GI= 22 (Low); Serving size= 1 cup sliced (121 g); GL= 0.6 (Low); Net carb= 2.7 g

Mushrooms Shiitake Stir-Fried ☛ GI= 22 (Low); Serving size= 1 cup whole (89 g); GL= 0.8 (Low); Net carb= 3.6 g

Mushrooms Stuffed ☛ GI= 22 (Low); Serving size= 1 stuffed cap (24 g); GL= 1.3 (Low); Net carb= 6 g

Mustard Cabbage—Cooked—(cooked with fat) ☛ GI= 32 (Low); Serving size= 1 cup (175 g); GL= 0.4 (Low); Net carb= 1.3 g

Mustard Cabbage—Cooked—(cooked without fat) ☛ GI= 32 (Low); Serving size= 1 cup (170 g); GL= 0.4 (Low); Net carb= 1.3 g

Mustard Greens ☛ GI= 33 (Low); Serving size= 1 cup, chopped (56 g); GL= 0.3 (Low); Net carb= 0.8 g

Mustard Greens—Cooked From Canned—(cooked without fat) ☛ GI= 33 (Low); Serving size= 1 cup, canned (153 g); GL= 1.3 (Low); Net carb= 3.8 g

Mustard Greens—Cooked From Canned—Made With Butter ☛ GI= 33 (Low); Serving size= 1 cup, canned (158 g); GL= 1.3 (Low); Net carb= 3.9 g

Mustard Greens—Cooked From Canned—Made With Oil ☛ GI= 33 (Low); Serving size= 1 cup, canned (158 g); GL= 1.3 (Low); Net carb= 3.9 g

Mustard Greens—Cooked From Fresh—(cooked without fat) ☛ GI= 33 (Low); Serving size= 1 cup, fresh (140 g); GL= 1.1 (Low); Net carb= 3.5 g

Mustard Greens—Cooked From Fresh—Made With Butter ☛ GI= 33 (Low); Serving size= 1 cup, fresh (145 g); GL= 1.2 (Low); Net carb= 3.5 g

Mustard Greens—Cooked From Fresh—Made With Oil ☛ GI= 33 (Low); Serving size= 1 cup, fresh (145 g); GL= 1.2 (Low); Net carb= 3.5 g

Mustard Greens—Cooked From Frozen—(cooked without fat) ☛ GI=

33 (Low); Serving size= 1 cup, frozen (150 g); GL= 0.1 (Low); Net carb= 0.4 g

Mustard Greens—Cooked From Frozen—Made With Butter ☛ GI= 33 (Low); Serving size= 1 cup, frozen (155 g); GL= 0.2 (Low); Net carb= 0.5 g

Mustard Greens—Cooked From Frozen—Made With Oil ☛ GI= 33 (Low); Serving size= 1 cup, frozen (155 g); GL= 0.2 (Low); Net carb= 0.5 g

Mustard Greens—Frozen—Unprepared ☛ GI= 32 (Low); Serving size= 1 cup, chopped (146 g); GL= 0.1 (Low); Net carb= 0.2 g

Mustard Spinach ☛ GI= 32 (Low); Serving size= 1 cup, chopped (150 g); GL= 0.5 (Low); Net carb= 1.7 g

New Zealand Spinach ☛ GI= 33 (Low); Serving size= 1 cup, chopped (56 g); GL= 0.2 (Low); Net carb= 0.6 g

Nopales ☛ GI= 35 (Low); Serving size= 1 cup, sliced (86 g); GL= 0.3 (Low); Net carb= 1 g

Okra ☛ GI= 32 (Low); Serving size= 1 cup (100 g); GL= 1.4 (Low); Net carb= 4.3 g

Okra Batter-Dipped Fried ☛ GI= 32 (Low); Serving size= 1 cup (92 g); GL= 6.4 (Low); Net carb= 20.1 g

Okra—Cooked—From Canned—(cooked without fat) ☛ GI= 32 (Low); Serving size= 1 cup (167 g); GL= 1.1 (Low); Net carb= 3.3 g

Okra—Cooked—From Canned—Made With Butter ☛ GI= 32 (Low); Serving size= 1 cup (172 g); GL= 1.1 (Low); Net carb= 3.4 g

Okra—Cooked—From Canned—Made With Oil ☛ GI= 32 (Low); Serving size= 1 cup (172 g); GL= 1.1 (Low); Net carb= 3.4 g

Okra—Cooked—From Fresh—(cooked without fat) ☛ GI= 32 (Low); Serving size= 1 cup (160 g); GL= 1 (Low); Net carb= 3.2 g

Okra—Cooked—From Fresh—Made With Butter ☛ GI= 32 (Low); Serving size= 1 cup (165 g); GL= 1 (Low); Net carb= 3.2 g

Okra—Cooked—From Fresh—Made With Oil ☛ GI= 32 (Low); Serving size= 1 cup (165 g); GL= 1 (Low); Net carb= 3.2 g

Okra—Cooked—From Frozen—(cooked without fat) ☛ GI= 32 (Low); Serving size= 1 cup (184 g); GL= 2.5 (Low); Net carb= 7.9 g

Okra—Cooked—From Frozen—Made With Butter ☛ GI= 32 (Low); Serving size= 1 cup (189 g); GL= 2.6 (Low); Net carb= 8 g

Okra—Cooked—From Frozen—Made With Oil ☛ GI= 32 (Low); Serving size= 1 cup (189 g); GL= 2.6 (Low); Net carb= 8 g

Okra Frozen—Unprepared ☛ GI= 32 (Low); Serving size= 1/3 package (10 oz) (95 g); GL= 1.3 (Low); Net carb= 4.2 g

Onions ☛ GI= 15 (Low); Serving size= 1 cup, chopped (160 g); GL= 1.8 (Low); Net carb= 12.2 g

Onions Canned—Solids And Liquids ☛ GI= 15 (Low); Serving size= 1 onion (63 g); GL= 0.3 (Low); Net carb= 1.8 g

Onions—Cooked—From Fresh—(cooked without fat) ☛ GI= 15 (Low); Serving size= 1 cup (210 g); GL= 2.7 (Low); Net carb= 18.3 g

Onions—Cooked—From Fresh—Made With Butter ☛ GI= 15 (Low); Serving size= 1 cup (210 g); GL= 2.7 (Low); Net carb= 17.8 g

Onions—Cooked—From Fresh—Made With Oil ☛ GI= 15 (Low); Serving size= 1 cup (210 g); GL= 2.7 (Low); Net carb= 17.8 g

Onions—Cooked—From Frozen—(cooked without fat) ☛ GI= 15 (Low); Serving size= 1 cup (210 g); GL= 1.5 (Low); Net carb= 10 g

Onions—Cooked—From Frozen—Made With Butter ☛ GI= 15 (Low); Serving size= 1 cup (215 g); GL= 1.5 (Low); Net carb= 9.9 g

Onions—Cooked—From Frozen—Made With Oil ☛ GI= 15 (Low); Serving size= 1 cup (215 g); GL= 1.5 (Low); Net carb= 9.9 g

Onions Dehydrated Flakes ☛ GI= 15 (Low); Serving size= 1 tbsp (5 g); GL= 0.6 (Low); Net carb= 3.7 g

Onions From Fresh—Creamed ☛ GI= 15 (Low); Serving size= 1 cup (228 g); GL= 3 (Low); Net carb= 20 g

Onions Frozen—Chopped Unprepared ☛ GI= 15 (Low); Serving size= 1/3 package (10 oz) (95 g); GL= 0.7 (Low); Net carb= 4.8 g

Onions Frozen—Whole Unprepared ☛ GI= 15 (Low); Serving size= 1/3 package (10 oz) (95 g); GL= 1 (Low); Net carb= 6.4 g

Onions Green—Cooked—From Fresh—(cooked with fat) ☛ GI= 15 (Low); Serving size= 1 cup (224 g); GL= 1.6 (Low); Net carb= 10.9 g

Onions Green—Cooked—From Fresh—(cooked without fat) ☛ GI= 15 (Low); Serving size= 1 cup (219 g); GL= 1.6 (Low); Net carb= 10.8 g

Onions Pearl—Cooked—From Canned ☛ GI= 15 (Low); Serving size= 1 cup (185 g); GL= 2.4 (Low); Net carb= 16.1 g

Onions Pearl—Cooked—From Fresh ☛ GI= 15 (Low); Serving size= 1 cup (185 g); GL= 2.4 (Low); Net carb= 16.1 g

Onions Pearl—Cooked—From Frozen ☛ GI= 15 (Low); Serving size= 1 cup (185 g); GL= 1.5 (Low); Net carb= 9.7 g

Onions Young Green Tops Only ☛ GI= 15 (Low); Serving size= 1 tbsp (6 g); GL= 0 (Low); Net carb= 0.2 g

Oriental Radishes ☛ GI= 32 (Low); Serving size= 1 cup slices (116 g); GL= 1.2 (Low); Net carb= 3.7 g

Oyster Mushrooms ☛ GI= 24 (Low); Serving size= 1 large (148 g); GL= 1.5 (Low); Net carb= 6.4 g

Pak-Choi (Bok Choy) (Cooked) ☛ GI= 32 (Low); Serving size= 1 cup, shredded (170 g); GL= 0.4 (Low); Net carb= 1.1 g

Palm Hearts (Canned) ☛ GI= 38 (Low); Serving size= 1 cup (146 g); GL= 1.2 (Low); Net carb= 3.2 g

Parsley ☛ GI= 32 (Low); Serving size= 1 cup chopped (60 g); GL= 0.6 (Low); Net carb= 1.8 g

Parsnips ☛ GI= 48 (Low); Serving size= 1 cup slices (133 g); GL= 8.4 (Low); Net carb= 17.4 g

Parsnips—Cooked—(cooked without fat) ☛ GI= 48 (Low); Serving size= 1 cup, pieces (156 g); GL= 10 (Low); Net carb= 20.7 g

Parsnips—Cooked—Made With Butter ☛ GI= 48 (Low); Serving size= 1 cup, pieces (161 g); GL= 10 (Low); Net carb= 20.8 g

Parsnips—Cooked—Made With Oil ☛ GI= 48 (Low); Serving size= 1 cup, pieces (161 g); GL= 10 (Low); Net carb= 20.8 g

Peas and Carrots—canned, low sodium, without fat ☛ GI= 48 (Low); Serving size= 1 cup (155 g); GL= 3.8 (Low); Net carb= 8 g

Peas and Carrots—cooked, from canned, without fat ☛ GI= 48 (Low); Serving size= 1 cup (155 g); GL= 4.8 (Low); Net carb= 10 g

Peas and Carrots—cooked, from fresh, without fat ☛ GI= 48 (Low); Serving size= 1 cup (155 g); GL= 3.8 (Low); Net carb= 8.1 g

Peas and Carrots—cooked—From Frozen, without fat ☛ GI= 48 (Low); Serving size= 1 cup (155 g); GL= 3.9 (Low); Net carb= 8.3 g

Peas and corn—cooked, without fat ☛ GI= 51 (Low); Serving size= 1 cup (155 g); GL= 4.1 (Low); Net carb= 8.1 g

Peas and Onions—cooked, without fat ☛ GI= 40 (Low); Serving size= 1 cup (155 g); GL= 8.7 (Low); Net carb= 21.7 g

Peas with Mushrooms—cooked, without fat ☛ GI= 47 (Low); Serving size= 1 cup (155 g); GL= 5.4 (Low); Net carb= 11.6 g

Peas, green—canned, low sodium, without fat ☛ GI= 48 (Low); Serving size= 1 cup (175 g); GL= 9.9 (Low); Net carb= 20.7 g

Peas, green—cooked, from canned, without fat ☛ GI= 48 (Low); Serving size= 1 cup (175 g); GL= 8.3 (Low); Net carb= 17.3 g

Peas, green—cooked, from fresh, without fat ☛ GI= 48 (Low); Serving size= 1 cup (175 g); GL= 8.4 (Low); Net carb= 17.6 g

Peas, green—cooked—From Frozen, without fat ☛ GI= 48 (Low); Serving size= 1 cup (175 g); GL= 8.3 (Low); Net carb= 17.2 g

Peas, green—raw ☛ GI= 48 (Low); Serving size= 1 cup (175 g); GL= 8.3 (Low); Net carb= 17.3 g

Pepper—green, cooked, without fat ☛ GI= 32 (Low); Serving size= 1 cup (115 g); GL= 2 (Low); Net carb= 6.3 g

Pepper—hot chili, raw ☛ GI= 32 (Low); Serving size= 1 pepper (73 g); GL= 0.9 (Low); Net carb= 2.8 g

Pepper—hot, cooked, from canned, with fat ☛ GI= 32 (Low); Serving size= 1 pepper (73 g); GL= 0.9 (Low); Net carb= 2.8 g

Pepper—hot, cooked, from canned, without fat ☛ GI= 32 (Low); Serving size= 1 pepper (73 g); GL= 0.9 (Low); Net carb= 2.8 g

Pepper—hot, cooked, from fresh, with fat ☛ GI= 32 (Low); Serving size= 1 pepper (73 g); GL= 0.9 (Low); Net carb= 2.8 g

Pepper—hot, cooked, from fresh, without fat ☛ GI= 32 (Low); Serving size= 1 pepper (73 g); GL= 0.9 (Low); Net carb= 2.8 g

Pepper—hot, cooked—From Frozen, without fat ☛ GI= 32 (Low); Serving size= 1 pepper (73 g); GL= 0.9 (Low); Net carb= 2.8 g

Pepper—hot, pickled ☛ GI= 32 (Low); Serving size= 1 pepper (73 g); GL= 0.9 (Low); Net carb= 2.8 g

Pepper—pickled ☛ GI= 32 (Low); Serving size= 1 pepper (73 g); GL= 0.9 (Low); Net carb= 2.8 g

Pepper—poblano, raw ☛ GI= 32 (Low); Serving size= 1 pepper (73 g); GL= 0.9 (Low); Net carb= 2.8 g

Pepper—red, cooked, without fat ☛ GI= 32 (Low); Serving size= 1 cup (110 g); GL= 3.9 (Low); Net carb= 12.1 g

Pepper—Serrano, raw ☛ GI= 32 (Low); Serving size= 1 cup (110 g); GL= 4.2 (Low); Net carb= 13.2 g

Pepper—sweet, green, raw ☛ GI= 32 (Low); Serving size= 1 cup (110 g); GL= 4.1 (Low); Net carb= 12.9 g

Pepper—sweet, red, raw ☛ GI= 32 (Low); Serving size= 1 cup (110 g); GL= 4.2 (Low); Net carb= 13 g

Pigeon peas—cooked ☛ GI= 22 (Low); Serving size= 1 cup (125 g); GL= 3.6 (Low); Net carb= 16.3 g

Pimiento ☛ GI= 32 (Low); Serving size= 1 cup (185 g); GL= 4.7 (Low); Net carb= 14.8 g

Radish—common, raw ☛ GI= 32 (Low); Serving size= 1 cup slices (116 g); GL= 1.9 (Low); Net carb= 5.9 g

Radish—Japanese (daikon), cooked, without fat ☛ GI= 32 (Low); Serving size= 1 cup slices (116 g); GL= 1.9 (Low); Net carb= 5.9 g

Radish—raw ☛ GI= 32 (Low); Serving size= 1 cup slices (116 g); GL= 1.2 (Low); Net carb= 3.7 g

Romaine Lettuce ☛ GI= 32 (Low); Serving size= 1 cup shredded (47 g); GL= 0.2 (Low); Net carb= 0.6 g

Rutabaga—Cooked—(cooked without fat) ☛ GI= 72 (High); Serving size= 1 cup, pieces (170 g); GL= 6.1 (Low); Net carb= 8.5 g

Rutabaga—Cooked—Made With Butter ☛ GI= 72 (High); Serving size= 1 cup, pieces (175 g); GL= 6.2 (Low); Net carb= 8.6 g

Rutabaga—Cooked—Made With Oil ☛ GI= 72 (High); Serving size= 1 cup, pieces (175 g); GL= 6.2 (Low); Net carb= 8.6 g

Rutabagas (Neeps Swedes) ☛ GI= 72 (High); Serving size= 1 cup, cubes (140 g); GL= 6.4 (Low); Net carb= 8.8 g

Salsify (Vegetable Oyster) Raw ☛ GI= 30 (Low); Serving size= 1 cup slices (133 g); GL= 6.1 (Low); Net carb= 20.3 g

Salsify—Cooked—(cooked with fat) ☛ GI= 30 (Low); Serving size= 1 cup (140 g); GL= 4.9 (Low); Net carb= 16.5 g

Salsify—Cooked—(cooked without fat) ☛ GI= 30 (Low); Serving size= 1 cup (135 g); GL= 4.9 (Low); Net carb= 16.4 g

Sauerkraut ☛ GI= 32 (Low); Serving size= 1 cup (142 g); GL= 0.6 (Low); Net carb= 2 g

Sauerkraut—canned ☛ GI= 32 (Low); Serving size= 1 cup (142 g); GL= 0.7 (Low); Net carb= 2.1 g

Sauerkraut—cooked, with fat ☛ GI= 32 (Low); Serving size= 1 cup (142 g); GL= 0.8 (Low); Net carb= 2.4 g

Sauerkraut—cooked, without fat ☛ GI= 32 (Low); Serving size= 1 cup (142 g); GL= 0.8 (Low); Net carb= 2.6 g

Sauteed Green Bell Peppers ☛ GI= 22 (Low); Serving size= 1 cup chopped (115 g); GL= 0.6 (Low); Net carb= 2.8 g

Savoy Cabbage ☛ GI= 32 (Low); Serving size= 1 cup, shredded (70 g); GL= 0.7 (Low); Net carb= 2.1 g

Scallop Squash ☛ GI= 48 (Low); Serving size= 1 cup slices (130 g); GL= 1.6 (Low); Net carb= 3.4 g

Seaweed Agar Raw ☛ GI= 48 (Low); Serving size= 2 tbsp (1/8 cup) (10 g); GL= 0.3 (Low); Net carb= 0.6 g

Snow Peas ☛ GI= 30 (Low); Serving size= 1 cup, chopped (98 g); GL= 1.5 (Low); Net carb= 4.9 g

Snowpea—Cooked—From Fresh—(cooked without fat) ☛ GI= 30 (Low); Serving size= 1 cup (160 g); GL= 2 (Low); Net carb= 6.7 g

Snowpea—Cooked—From Fresh—Made With Butter ☛ GI= 30 (Low); Serving size= 1 cup (165 g); GL= 2 (Low); Net carb= 6.8 g

Soybean Sprouts ☛ GI= 15 (Low); Serving size= 1/2 cup (35 g); GL= 0.4 (Low); Net carb= 3 g

Spaghetti Squash ☛ GI= 20 (Low); Serving size= 1 cup, cubes (101 g); GL= 1.1 (Low); Net carb= 5.4 g

Spinach ☛ GI= 18 (Low); Serving size= 1 cup (30 g); GL= 0.1 (Low); Net carb= 0.4 g

Spinach And Cheese Casserole ☛ GI= 18 (Low); Serving size= 1 cup (200 g); GL= 2.6 (Low); Net carb= 14.5 g

Spinach Canned—Regular Pack Drained Solids ☛ GI= 18 (Low); Serving size= 1 cup (214 g); GL= 0.4 (Low); Net carb= 2.1 g

Spinach Canned—Regular Pack Solids And Liquids ☛ GI= 18 (Low); Serving size= 1 cup (234 g); GL= 0.6 (Low); Net carb= 3.1 g

Spinach—Cooked—From Canned—(cooked without fat) ☛ GI= 18 (Low); Serving size= 1 cup, canned (214 g); GL= 0.4 (Low); Net carb= 2.2 g

Spinach—Cooked—From Canned—Made With Butter ☛ GI= 18 (Low); Serving size= 1 cup, canned (219 g); GL= 0.4 (Low); Net carb= 2.2 g

Spinach—Cooked—From Canned—Made With Oil ☛ GI= 18 (Low); Serving size= 1 cup, canned (219 g); GL= 0.4 (Low); Net carb= 2.2 g

Spring Onions ☛ GI= 15 (Low); Serving size= 1 cup, chopped (100 g); GL= 0.7 (Low); Net carb= 4.7 g

Squash Spaghetti—Cooked—(cooked without fat) ☛ GI= 20 (Low); Serving size= 1 cup, cooked (155 g); GL= 1.6 (Low); Net carb= 7.8 g

Squash Spaghetti—Cooked—Made With Butter ☛ GI= 20 (Low); Serving size= 1 cup, cooked (160 g); GL= 1.5 (Low); Net carb= 7.7 g

Squash Spaghetti—Cooked—Made With Oil ☛ GI= 20 (Low); Serving size= 1 cup, cooked (160 g); GL= 1.5 (Low); Net carb= 7.7 g

Squash Summer From Frozen—Creamed ☛ GI= 15 (Low); Serving size= 1 cup (217 g); GL= 1.7 (Low); Net carb= 11.6 g

Squash Summer Yellow Or Green Breaded Or Battered Baked ☛ GI= 15 (Low); Serving size= 1 cup (220 g); GL= 3.9 (Low); Net carb= 25.9 g

Squash Summer Yellow Or Green Breaded Or Battered Fried ☛ GI= 15 (Low); Serving size= 1 cup (220 g); GL= 3.7 (Low); Net carb= 24.8 g

Sun-Dried Tomatoes ☛ GI= 36 (Low); Serving size= 1 cup (54 g); GL= 8.4 (Low); Net carb= 23.5 g

Swamp Cabbage ☛ GI= 32 (Low); Serving size= 1 cup, chopped (56 g); GL= 0.2 (Low); Net carb= 0.6 g

Sweet Onions ☛ GI= 17 (Low); Serving size= 1 nlea serving (148 g); GL= 1.7 (Low); Net carb= 9.8 g

Sweet Pickled Relish ☛ GI= 32 (Low); Serving size= 1 tbsp (15 g); GL= 1.6 (Low); Net carb= 5.1 g

Sweet Potato Boiled (cooked without fat) ☛ GI= 66 (Medium); Serving size= 1 small (80 g); GL= 8.3 (Low); Net carb= 12.6 g

Sweet Potato Boiled Made With Butter ☛ GI= 66 (Medium); Serving size= 1 small (80 g); GL= 7.6 (Low); Net carb= 11.5 g

Sweet Potato Boiled Made With Oil ☛ GI= 66 (Medium); Serving size= 1 small (80 g); GL= 7.6 (Low); Net carb= 11.5 g

Swiss Chard ☛ GI= 32 (Low); Serving size= 1 cup (36 g); GL= 0.2 (Low); Net carb= 0.8 g

Taro ☛ GI= 32 (Low); Serving size= 1 cup, sliced (104 g); GL= 7.4 (Low); Net carb= 23.3 g

Taro Leaves Raw ☛ GI= 32 (Low); Serving size= 1 cup (28 g); GL= 0.3 (Low); Net carb= 0.8 g

Tomatillos ☛ GI= 38 (Low); Serving size= 1 medium (34 g); GL= 0.5 (Low); Net carb= 1.3 g

Tomatoes ☛ GI= 38 (Low); Serving size= 1 cup cherry tomatoes (149 g); GL= 1.5 (Low); Net carb= 4 g

Tomatoes Crushed Canned ☛ GI= 38 (Low); Serving size= 1/2 cup (121 g); GL= 2.5 (Low); Net carb= 6.5 g

Tomatoes From Fresh—Broiled ☛ GI= 38 (Low); Serving size= 1 cherry (14 g); GL= 0.2 (Low); Net carb= 0.5 g

Tomatoes From Fresh—Scalloped ☛ GI= 38 (Low); Serving size= 1 cup (235 g); GL= 8.4 (Low); Net carb= 22.2 g

Tomatoes From Fresh—Stewed ☛ GI= 38 (Low); Serving size= 1 tomato (114 g); GL= 3.8 (Low); Net carb= 9.9 g

Tomatoes Green—Cooked—From Fresh ☛ GI= 38 (Low); Serving size= 1 small (75 g); GL= 3.4 (Low); Net carb= 9 g

Tomatoes Orange Raw ☛ GI= 38 (Low); Serving size= 1 cup, chopped (158 g); GL= 1.4 (Low); Net carb= 3.6 g

Tomatoes Red From Fresh—Fried ☛ GI= 38 (Low); Serving size= 1 small (75 g); GL= 2.8 (Low); Net carb= 7.4 g

Tomatoes Sun-Dried Packed In Oil Drained ☛ GI= 38 (Low); Serving size= 1 cup (110 g); GL= 7.3 (Low); Net carb= 19.3 g

Turnip—Cooked—From Canned—(cooked without fat) ☛ GI= 32 (Low); Serving size= 1 cup, pieces (155 g); GL= 1.5 (Low); Net carb= 4.7 g

Turnip—Cooked—From Canned—Made With Butter ☛ GI= 32 (Low); Serving size= 1 cup, pieces (160 g); GL= 1.5 (Low); Net carb= 4.8 g

Turnip—Cooked—From Canned—Made With Oil ☛ GI= 32 (Low); Serving size= 1 cup, pieces (160 g); GL= 1.5 (Low); Net carb= 4.8 g

Turnip—Cooked—From Fresh—(cooked without fat) ☛ GI= 32 (Low); Serving size= 1 cup, pieces (155 g); GL= 1.6 (Low); Net carb= 4.8 g

Turnip—Cooked—From Fresh—Made With Butter ☛ GI= 32 (Low); Serving size= 1 cup, pieces (160 g); GL= 1.5 (Low); Net carb= 4.8 g

Turnip—Cooked—From Fresh—Made With Oil ☛ GI= 32 (Low); Serving size= 1 cup, pieces (160 g); GL= 1.5 (Low); Net carb= 4.8 g

Turnip—Cooked—From Frozen—(cooked without fat) ☛ GI= 32 (Low); Serving size= 1 cup, pieces (155 g); GL= 1.2 (Low); Net carb= 3.7 g

Turnip—Cooked—From Frozen—Made With Butter ☛ GI= 32 (Low); Serving size= 1 cup, pieces (160 g); GL= 1.2 (Low); Net carb= 3.7 g

Turnip—Cooked—From Frozen—Made With Oil ☛ GI= 32 (Low); Serving size= 1 cup, pieces (160 g); GL= 1.2 (Low); Net carb= 3.7 g

Turnip Greens ☛ GI= 32 (Low); Serving size= 1 cup, chopped (55 g); GL= 0.7 (Low); Net carb= 2.2 g

Turnips ☛ GI= 32 (Low); Serving size= 1 cup, cubes (130 g); GL= 1.9 (Low); Net carb= 6 g

Wakame ☛ GI= 50 (Low); Serving size= 2 tbsp (1/8 cup) (10 g); GL= 0.4 (Low); Net carb= 0.9 g

Wasabi Root ☛ GI= 41 (Low); Serving size= 1 cup, sliced (130 g); GL= 8.4 (Low); Net carb= 20.5 g

Waterchestnuts Chinese Raw ☛ GI= 54 (Low); Serving size= 1/2 cup slices (62 g); GL= 7 (Low); Net carb= 13 g

Waterchestnuts Chinese Canned—Solids And Liquids ☛ GI= 54 (Low); Serving size= 1/2 cup slices (70 g); GL= 3.7 (Low); Net carb= 6.9 g

Watercress ☛ GI= 32 (Low); Serving size= 1 cup, chopped (34 g); GL= 0.1 (Low); Net carb= 0.3 g

Watercress—Cooked—(cooked with fat) ☛ GI= 32 (Low); Serving size= 1 cup (142 g); GL= 0.3 (Low); Net carb= 1 g

Watercress—Cooked—(cooked without fat) ☛ GI= 32 (Low); Serving size= 1 cup (137 g); GL= 0.3 (Low); Net carb= 1.1 g

Winged Beans Immature Seeds Raw ☛ GI= 50 (Low); Serving size= 1 cup slices (44 g); GL= 0.9 (Low); Net carb= 1.9 g

Winter Squash ☛ GI= 51 (Low); Serving size= 1 cup, cubes (116 g); GL= 4.2 (Low); Net carb= 8.2 g

Yardlong Bean Raw ☛ GI= 82 (High); Serving size= 1 cup slices (91 g); GL= 6.2 (Low); Net carb= 7.6 g

Zucchini ☛ GI= 15 (Low); Serving size= 1 cup, chopped (124 g); GL= 0.4 (Low); Net carb= 2.6 g

PART VIII
THE WORST FOODS TO EAT (HIGH GLYCEMIC LOAD FOOD)

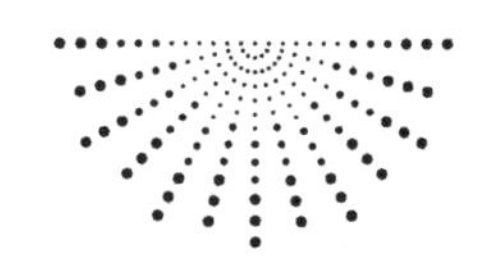

37
BAKED PRODUCTS

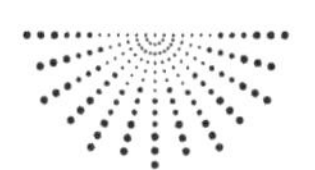

Basbousa ☛ Serving size= 1 piece (about 3 x 2-1/2"), 82 g; GI= 63 (Medium); GL= 25.5 (High); Net carb= 40.5 g

Biscuit—Plain Or Buttermilk Dry Mix ☛ Serving size= 1 cup, purchased, 120 g; GI= 70 (High); GL= 51.5 (High); Net carb= 73.6 g

Bread—Chapati Or Roti Plain ☛ Serving size= 1 piece, 68 g; GI= 81 (High); GL= 22.8 (High); Net carb= 28.2 g

Bread—French Or Vienna Whole Wheat ☛ Serving size= 1 slice 1 serving, 48 g; GI= 95 (High); GL= 20.5 (High); Net carb= 21.6 g

Brioche ☛ Serving size= 1 piece, 77 g; GI= 91 (High); GL= 24.1 (High); Net carb= 26.5 g

Cake Or Cupcake—German Chocolate With Icing Or Filling ☛ Serving size= 1 regular cupcake, 75 g; GI= 55 (Medium); GL= 20.1 (High); Net carb= 36.6 g

Cake Or Cupcake—Fruit With Icing Or Filling ☛ Serving size= 1 regular cupcake, 75 g; GI= 55 (Medium); GL= 22.6 (High); Net carb= 41 g

Cake Or Cupcake—Nut With Icing Or Filling ☛ Serving size= 1 regular cupcake, 75 g; GI= 55 (Medium); GL= 21.8 (High); Net carb= 39.7 g

Cake—White Made From Recipe Without Frosting ☛ Serving size= 1 piece (1/12 of 9 inch dia), 74 g; GI= 55 (Medium); GL= 22.9 (High); Net carb= 41.7 g

Cake—Yellow Enriched Dry Mix ☛ Serving size= 1 serving, 43 g; GI= 55 (Medium); GL= 19.1 (High); Net carb= 34.7 g

Cake—Yellow Made From Recipe Without Frosting ☛ Serving size= 1 piece (1/12 of 8 inch dia), 68 g; GI= 55 (Medium); GL= 19.6 (High); Net carb= 35.6 g

Cobbler—Apple ☛ Serving size= 1 cup, 217 g; GI= 67 (Medium); GL= 51.7 (High); Net carb= 77.2 g

Cobbler—Apricot ☛ Serving size= 1 cup, 217 g; GI= 67 (Medium); GL= 49.4 (High); Net carb= 73.7 g

Cobbler—Berry ☛ Serving size= 1 cup, 217 g; GI= 67 (Medium); GL= 60 (High); Net carb= 89.5 g

Cobbler—Cherry ☛ Serving size= 1 cup, 217 g; GI= 67 (Medium); GL= 50.3 (High); Net carb= 75.1 g

Cobbler—Peach ☛ Serving size= 1 cup, 217 g; GI= 67 (Medium); GL= 53.4 (High); Net carb= 79.7 g

Cobbler—Pear ☛ Serving size= 1 cup, 217 g; GI= 67 (Medium); GL= 57.8 (High); Net carb= 86.2 g

Cobbler—Pineapple ☛ Serving size= 1 cup, 217 g; GI= 67 (Medium); GL= 52.3 (High); Net carb= 78 g

Cobbler—Plum ☛ Serving size= 1 cup, 217 g; GI= 67 (Medium); GL= 53.9 (High); Net carb= 80.4 g

Cobbler—Rhubarb ☛ Serving size= 1 cup, 217 g; GI= 67 (Medium); GL= 66.3 (High); Net carb= 98.9 g

CornBread—Muffin Stick Round Made From Home Recipe ☛ Serving size= 1 small, 66 g; GI= 73 (High); GL= 21.3 (High); Net carb= 29.2 g

Cornmeal—Dumpling ☛ Serving size= 1 cup, cooked, 240 g; GI= 75 (High); GL= 43.7 (High); Net carb= 58.3 g

Cream Puff Eclair Custard ☛ Serving size= 4 oz, 113 g; GI= 59 (Medium); GL= 24.4 (High); Net carb= 41.3 g

Crisp Apple Apple Dessert ☛ Serving size= 1 cup, 246 g; GI= 61 (Medium); GL= 43.8 (High); Net carb= 71.8 g

Crisp Blueberry ☛ Serving size= 1 cup, 246 g; GI= 59 (Medium); GL= 57 (High); Net carb= 96.6 g

Crisp Cherry ☛ Serving size= 1 cup, 246 g; GI= 60 (Medium); GL= 68.2 (High); Net carb= 113.6 g

Crisp Peach ☛ Serving size= 1 cup, 246 g; GI= 63 (Medium); GL= 56.6 (High); Net carb= 89.8 g

Crisp Rhubarb ☛ Serving size= 1 cup, 246 g; GI= 59 (Medium); GL= 59.9 (High); Net carb= 101.5 g

Doughnut—Chocolate Cream-Filled ☛ Serving size= 1 doughnut, 65 g; GI= 75 (High); GL= 19.4 (High); Net carb= 25.9 g

Doughnut—Chocolate Raised Or Yeast With Chocolate Icing ☛ Serving size= 1 doughnut (3" dia), 71 g; GI= 78 (High); GL= 27.9 (High); Net carb= 35.8 g

Doughnut—Custard-Filled With Icing ☛ Serving size= 1 doughnut, 70 g; GI= 79 (High); GL= 30 (High); Net carb= 38 g

Doughnut—Raised Or Yeast Chocolate Covered ☛ Serving size= 1 doughnut (3" dia), 71 g; GI= 77 (High); GL= 27.5 (High); Net carb= 35.7 g

Dutch Apple Pie ☛ Serving size= 1/8 pie 1 pie (1/8 of 9 inch pie), 131 g; GI= 55 (Medium); GL= 31 (High); Net carb= 56.3 g

English Muffins—Whole Grain White ☛ Serving size= 1 muffin 1 serving, 57 g; GI= 77 (High); GL= 20.5 (High); Net carb= 26.6 g

Muffin—Chocolate Chip ☛ Serving size= 1 muffin, 58 g; GI= 63 (Medium); GL= 19.5 (High); Net carb= 31 g

Muffin—English Oat Bran With Raisins ☛ Serving size= 1 muffin, 58 g; GI= 70 (High); GL= 19.3 (High); Net carb= 27.6 g

Pie Crust—Cookie-Type Chocolate Ready Crust ☛ Serving size= 1 crust, 182 g; GI= 59 (Medium); GL= 66.3 (High); Net carb= 112.4 g

Pie Crust—Cookie-Type Made From Recipe Vanilla Wafer Chilled ☛ Serving size= 1 cup, 129 g; GI= 59 (Medium); GL= 38.1 (High); Net carb= 64.6 g

Pie Crust—Refrigerated Regular Baked ☛ Serving size= 1 pie crust, 198 g; GI= 59 (Medium); GL= 66.7 (High); Net carb= 113.1 g

Pie—Apple Diet ☛ Serving size= 1 individual serving, 85 g; GI= 59 (Medium); GL= 21.4 (High); Net carb= 36.2 g

Pie—Banana Cream Individual Size Or Tart ☛ Serving size= 1 tart, 117 g; GI= 59 (Medium); GL= 20.7 (High); Net carb= 35 g

Pie—Berry, Individual Size Or Tart ☛ Serving size= 1 tart, 117 g; GI= 59 (Medium); GL= 26.6 (High); Net carb= 45.1 g

Pie—Blackberry Individual Size Or Tart ☛ Serving size= 1 tart, 117 g; GI= 59 (Medium); GL= 23.4 (High); Net carb= 39.7 g

Pie—Blueberry Individual Size Or Tart ☛ Serving size= 1 tart, 117 g; GI= 59 (Medium); GL= 25.5 (High); Net carb= 43.3 g

Pie—Chocolate Cream Individual Size Or Tart ☛ Serving size= 1 tart, 117 g; GI= 59 (Medium); GL= 24 (High); Net carb= 40.6 g

Pie—Chocolate Creme Commercially Made ☛ Serving size= 1 serving .167 pie, 120 g; GI= 59 (Medium); GL= 26.7 (High); Net carb= 45.2 g

Pie—Peach Individual Size Or Tart ☛ Serving size= 1 tart, 117 g; GI= 59 (Medium); GL= 26 (High); Net carb= 44.1 g

Pie—Pear Individual Size Or Tart ☛ Serving size= 1 tart, 117 g; GI= 59 (Medium); GL= 25.6 (High); Net carb= 43.4 g

Pie—Pudding Chocolate, Individual Size, With Chocolate Coating ☛ Serving size= 1 individual pie, 142 g; GI= 59 (Medium); GL= 34.3 (High); Net carb= 58.2 g

Pie—Pudding Flavors, Individual Size or Tart, Other Than Chocolate ☛ Serving size= 1 small tart, 117 g; GI= 59 (Medium); GL= 26.1 (High); Net carb= 44.3 g

Pie—Raisin Individual Size Or Tart ☛ Serving size= 1 tart, 117 g; GI= 59 (Medium); GL= 27 (High); Net carb= 45.8 g

Pie—Rhubarb Individual Size Or Tart ☛ Serving size= 1 tart, 117 g; GI= 59 (Medium); GL= 25.1 (High); Net carb= 42.5 g

Pie—Strawberry Cream Individual Size Or Tart ☛ Serving size= 1 tart, 117 g; GI= 59 (Medium); GL= 19.1 (High); Net carb= 32.3 g

Pie—Strawberry Individual Size Or Tart ☛ Serving size= 1 tart, 117 g; GI= 59 (Medium); GL= 23.9 (High); Net carb= 40.5 g

Pizza Cheese And Vegetables Gluten-Free—Thick Crust ☛ Serving size= 1 piece, nfs, 149 g; GI= 61 (Medium); GL= 21.4 (High); Net carb= 35.1 g

Pizza—Cheese And Vegetables Whole Wheat—Thick Crust ☛ Serving size= 1 piece, nfs, 149 g; GI= 62 (Medium); GL= 23.2 (High); Net carb= 37.4 g

Pizza—Cheese From School Lunch Medium Crust ☛ Serving size= 1 piece, nfs, 147 g; GI= 63 (Medium); GL= 24.4 (High); Net carb= 38.7 g

Pizza—Cheese Gluten-Free—Thick Crust ☛ Serving size= 1 piece, nfs, 132 g; GI= 63 (Medium); GL= 22.6 (High); Net carb= 35.8 g

Pizza—Cheese Whole Wheat—Thick Crust ☛ Serving size= 1 piece, nfs, 132 g; GI= 64 (Medium); GL= 24.5 (High); Net carb= 38.3 g

Pizza—Cheese With Fruit Medium Crust ☛ Serving size= 1 piece, nfs, 137 g; GI= 64 (Medium); GL= 25.3 (High); Net carb= 39.5 g

Pizza—Cheese With Fruit—Thick Crust ☛ Serving size= 1 piece, nfs, 150 g; GI= 64 (Medium); GL= 27.8 (High); Net carb= 43.4 g

Pizza—Cheese With Vegetables From Frozen—Thick Crust ☛ Serving size= 1 piece, nfs, 143 g; GI= 64 (Medium); GL= 26.4 (High); Net carb= 41.3 g

Pizza—Cheese With Vegetables From Restaurant Or Fast Food Medium Crust ☛ Serving size= 1 piece, nfs, 133 g; GI= 64 (Medium); GL= 24.3 (High); Net carb= 37.9 g

Pizza—Cheese With Vegetables From Restaurant Or Fast Food—Thick Crust ☛ Serving size= 1 piece, nfs, 149 g; GI= 64 (Medium); GL= 27 (High); Net carb= 42.2 g

Pizza—Extra Cheese—Thick Crust ☛ Serving size= 1 piece, nfs, 141 g; GI= 65 (Medium); GL= 27.3 (High); Net carb= 42 g

Pizza—No Cheese—Thick Crust ☛ Serving size= 1 piece, nfs, 124 g; GI= 73 (High); GL= 32.5 (High); Net carb= 44.5 g

Pizza—Rolls ☛ Serving size= 1 cup, 119 g; GI= 80 (High); GL= 49.6 (High); Net carb= 62 g

Roll—Sweet Frosted ☛ Serving size= 1 small, 54 g; GI= 77 (High); GL= 20.1 (High); Net carb= 26.1 g

Roll—Sweet With Fruit Frosted ☛ Serving size= 1 small, 54 g; GI= 77 (High); GL= 21.4 (High); Net carb= 27.8 g

Waffle—Chocolate Chip Frozen—Ready-To-Heat ☛ Serving size= 2 waffles, 70 g; GI= 76 (High); GL= 23.5 (High); Net carb= 30.9 g

Waffle—Whole Wheat Lowfat Frozen—Ready-To-Heat ☛ Serving size= 1 serving 2 waffles, 70 g; GI= 72 (High); GL= 22.6 (High); Net carb= 31.4 g

38
BEEF, LAMP, VEAL, PORK & POULTRY

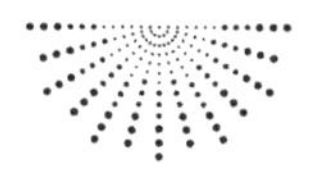

Beef-Offal—Heart: Breaded + fried ☛ Serving size= 3 oz, 85 g; GI= 95 (High); GL= 20 (High); Net carb= 21 g

Beef—Bottom Round: Breaded + fried ☛ Serving size= 3 oz, 85 g; GI= 95 (High); GL= 20 (High); Net carb= 21 g

Beef—Brain: Breaded + fried ☛ Serving size= 3 oz, 85 g; GI= 95 (High); GL= 20 (High); Net carb= 21 g

Beef—Brisket: Breaded + fried ☛ Serving size= 3 oz, 85 g; GI= 95 (High); GL= 20 (High); Net carb= 21 g

Beef—Chuck Roast: Breaded + fried ☛ Serving size= 3 oz, 85 g; GI= 95 (High); GL= 20 (High); Net carb= 21 g

Beef—Chuck Steak Varieties Chart: Breaded + fried ☛ Serving size= 3 oz, 85 g; GI= 95 (High); GL= 20 (High); Net carb= 21 g

Beef—Cuts of Steak: Breaded + fried ☛ Serving size= 3 oz, 85 g; GI= 95 (High); GL= 20 (High); Net carb= 21 g

Beef—Delmonico Steak: Breaded + fried ☛ Serving size= 3 oz, 85 g; GI= 95 (High); GL= 20 (High); Net carb= 21 g

Beef—Hanger Steak: Breaded + fried ☛ Serving size= 3 oz, 85 g; GI= 95 (High); GL= 20 (High); Net carb= 21 g

Beef—Kidney: Breaded + fried ☛ Serving size= 1 slice, 81 g; GI= 95 (High); GL= 20 (High); Net carb= 21 g

Beef—Liver: Battered + fried ☛ Serving size= 1 slice, 81 g; GI= 95 (High); GL= 20 (High); Net carb= 21.1 g

Beef—Liver: Breaded + fried ☛ Serving size= 1 slice, 81 g; GI= 95 (High); GL= 23.8 (High); Net carb= 25.1 g

Beef—Loin Steaks and/or Steak Types: Breaded + fried ☛ Serving size= 3 oz, 85 g; GI= 95 (High); GL= 20 (High); Net carb= 21 g

Beef—Mock Tender Petite Fillet: Breaded + fried ☛ Serving size= 3 oz, 85 g; GI= 95 (High); GL= 20 (High); Net carb= 21 g

Beef—Prime Rib: Breaded + fried ☛ Serving size= 3 oz, 85 g; GI= 95 (High); GL= 20 (High); Net carb= 21 g

Beef—Rib Steak Cuts: Breaded + fried ☛ Serving size= 3 oz, 85 g; GI= 95 (High); GL= 20 (High); Net carb= 21 g

Beef—Round Steak Varieties: Breaded + fried ☛ Serving size= 3 oz, 85 g; GI= 95 (High); GL= 20 (High); Net carb= 21 g

Beef—Short Loin: Breaded + fried ☛ Serving size= 3 oz, 85 g; GI= 95 (High); GL= 20 (High); Net carb= 21 g

Beef—Short Ribs: Breaded + fried ☛ Serving size= 3 oz, 85 g; GI= 95 (High); GL= 20 (High); Net carb= 21 g

Beef—T-Bone Steak: Breaded + fried ☛ Serving size= 3 oz, 85 g; GI= 95 (High); GL= 20 (High); Net carb= 21 g

Beef—Tenderloin: Breaded + fried ☛ Serving size= 3 oz, 85 g; GI= 95 (High); GL= 20 (High); Net carb= 21 g

Beef—Tongue: Breaded + fried ☛ Serving size= 1 slice, 81 g; GI= 95 (High); GL= 20 (High); Net carb= 21 g

Beef—Top Sirloin: Breaded + fried ☛ Serving size= 3 oz, 85 g; GI= 95 (High); GL= 20 (High); Net carb= 21 g

Beef—Tri-Tip: Breaded + fried ☛ Serving size= 3 oz, 85 g; GI= 95 (High); GL= 20 (High); Net carb= 21 g

Beef—Tripe: Breaded + fried ☛ Serving size= 1 slice, 81 g; GI= 95 (High); GL= 20 (High); Net carb= 21 g

Chicken—Backs and Necks: Breaded + fried ☛ Serving size= 3 oz, 85 g; GI= 95 (High); GL= 20 (High); Net carb= 21 g

Chicken—Breast Fillet Tenderloin: Breaded + fried ☛ Serving size= 3 oz, 85 g; GI= 95 (High); GL= 20 (High); Net carb= 21 g

Chicken—Drumstick: Breaded + fried ☛ Serving size= 3 oz, 85 g; GI= 95 (High); GL= 20 (High); Net carb= 21 g

Chicken—Leg: Breaded + fried ☛ Serving size= 3 oz, 85 g; GI= 95 (High); GL= 20 (High); Net carb= 21 g

Chicken—Tender: Breaded + fried ☛ Serving size= 3 oz, 85 g; GI= 95 (High); GL= 20 (High); Net carb= 21 g

Chicken—Thigh: Breaded + fried ☛ Serving size= 3 oz, 85 g; GI= 95 (High); GL= 20 (High); Net carb= 21 g

Chicken—Wing: Breaded + fried ☛ Serving size= 3 oz, 85 g; GI= 95 (High); GL= 20 (High); Net carb= 21 g

Lamb—Breast: Breaded + fried ☛ Serving size= 3 oz, 85 g; GI= 95 (High); GL= 20 (High); Net carb= 21 g

Lamb—Cutlets: Breaded + fried ☛ Serving size= 3 oz, 85 g; GI= 95 (High); GL= 20 (High); Net carb= 21 g

Lamb—Leg: Breaded + fried ☛ Serving size= 3 oz, 85 g; GI= 95 (High); GL= 20 (High); Net carb= 21 g

Lamb—Loin: Breaded + fried ☛ Serving size= 3 oz, 85 g; GI= 95 (High); GL= 20 (High); Net carb= 21 g

Lamb—Neck: Breaded + fried ☛ Serving size= 3 oz, 85 g; GI= 95 (High); GL= 20 (High); Net carb= 21 g

Lamb—Rack: Breaded + fried ☛ Serving size= 3 oz, 85 g; GI= 95 (High); GL= 20 (High); Net carb= 21 g

Lamb—Rump: Breaded + fried ☛ Serving size= 3 oz, 85 g; GI= 95 (High); GL= 20 (High); Net carb= 21 g

Lamb—Shank: Breaded + fried ☛ Serving size= 3 oz, 85 g; GI= 95 (High); GL= 20 (High); Net carb= 21 g

Lamb—Shoulder: Breaded + fried ☛ Serving size= 3 oz, 85 g; GI= 95 (High); GL= 20 (High); Net carb= 21 g

Pork—back ribs: Breaded + fried ☛ Serving size= 3 oz, 85 g; GI= 95 (High); GL= 20 (High); Net carb= 21 g

Pork—Belly: Breaded + fried ☛ Serving size= 3 oz, 85 g; GI= 95 (High); GL= 20 (High); Net carb= 21 g

Pork—Cutlets: Breaded + fried ☛ Serving size= 3 oz, 85 g; GI= 95 (High); GL= 20 (High); Net carb= 21 g

Pork—Garlic Sausages: Breaded + fried ☛ Serving size= 3 oz, 85 g; GI= 95 (High); GL= 20 (High); Net carb= 21 g

Pork—Ham: Breaded + fried ☛ Serving size= 3 oz, 85 g; GI= 95 (High); GL= 20 (High); Net carb= 21 g

Pork—Loin: Breaded + fried ☛ Serving size= 3 oz, 85 g; GI= 95 (High); GL= 20 (High); Net carb= 21 g

Pork—Rib chops: Breaded + fried ☛ Serving size= 3 oz, 85 g; GI= 95 (High); GL= 20 (High); Net carb= 21 g

Pork—Roasts: Breaded + fried ☛ Serving size= 3 oz, 85 g; GI= 95 (High); GL= 20 (High); Net carb= 21 g

Pork—Sausages: Breaded + fried ☛ Serving size= 3 oz, 85 g; GI= 95 (High); GL= 20 (High); Net carb= 21 g

Pork—Shoulder chops: Breaded + fried ☛ Serving size= 3 oz, 85 g; GI= 95 (High); GL= 20 (High); Net carb= 21 g

Pork—Sirloin chops: Breaded + fried ☛ Serving size= 3 oz, 85 g; GI= 95 (High); GL= 20 (High); Net carb= 21 g

Pork—spare ribs: Breaded + fried ☛ Serving size= 3 oz, 85 g; GI= 95 (High); GL= 20 (High); Net carb= 21 g

Turkey—Backs and Necks: Breaded + fried ☛ Serving size= 3 oz, 85 g; GI= 95 (High); GL= 20 (High); Net carb= 21 g

Turkey—Breast Fillet Tenderloin: Breaded + fried ☛ Serving size= 3 oz, 85 g; GI= 95 (High); GL= 20 (High); Net carb= 21 g

Turkey—Breast: Breaded + fried ☛ Serving size= 3 oz, 85 g; GI= 95 (High); GL= 20 (High); Net carb= 21 g

Turkey—Drumstick: Breaded + fried ☛ Serving size= 3 oz, 85 g; GI= 95 (High); GL= 20 (High); Net carb= 21 g

Turkey—Leg: Breaded + fried ☛ Serving size= 3 oz, 85 g; GI= 95 (High); GL= 20 (High); Net carb= 21 g

Turkey—Tender: Breaded + fried ☛ Serving size= 3 oz, 85 g; GI= 95 (High); GL= 20 (High); Net carb= 21 g

Turkey—Thigh: Breaded + fried ☛ Serving size= 3 oz, 85 g; GI= 95 (High); GL= 20 (High); Net carb= 21 g

Turkey—Wing: Breaded + fried ☛ Serving size= 3 oz, 85 g; GI= 95 (High); GL= 20 (High); Net carb= 21 g

Veal-Offal—Heart: Breaded + fried ☛ Serving size= 3 oz, 85 g; GI= 95 (High); GL= 20 (High); Net carb= 21 g

Veal—Bottom Round: Breaded + fried ☛ Serving size= 3 oz, 85 g; GI= 95 (High); GL= 20 (High); Net carb= 21 g

Veal—Brain: Breaded + fried ☛ Serving size= 3 oz, 85 g; GI= 95 (High); GL= 20 (High); Net carb= 21 g

Veal—Brisket: Breaded + fried ☛ Serving size= 3 oz, 85 g; GI= 95 (High); GL= 20 (High); Net carb= 21 g

Veal—Chuck Roast: Breaded + fried ☛ Serving size= 3 oz, 85 g; GI= 95 (High); GL= 20 (High); Net carb= 21 g

Veal—Chuck Steak Varieties Chart: Breaded + fried ☛ Serving size= 3 oz, 85 g; GI= 95 (High); GL= 20 (High); Net carb= 21 g

Veal—Cuts of Steak: Breaded + fried ☛ Serving size= 3 oz, 85 g; GI= 95 (High); GL= 20 (High); Net carb= 21 g

Veal—Delmonico Steak: Breaded + fried ☛ Serving size= 3 oz, 85 g; GI= 95 (High); GL= 20 (High); Net carb= 21 g

Veal—Hanger Steak: Breaded + fried ☛ Serving size= 3 oz, 85 g; GI= 95 (High); GL= 20 (High); Net carb= 21 g

Veal—Kidney: Breaded + fried ☛ Serving size= 2 slice, 81 g; GI= 95 (High); GL= 20 (High); Net carb= 21 g

Veal—Liver: Battered + fried ☛ Serving size= 1 slice, 81 g; GI= 95 (High); GL= 20 (High); Net carb= 21.1 g

Veal—Liver: Breaded + fried ☛ Serving size= 1 slice, 81 g; GI= 95 (High); GL= 23.8 (High); Net carb= 25.1 g

Veal—Loin Steaks and/or Steak Types: Breaded + fried ☛ Serving size= 3 oz, 85 g; GI= 95 (High); GL= 20 (High); Net carb= 21 g

Veal—Mock Tender Petite Fillet: Breaded + fried ☛ Serving size= 3 oz, 85 g; GI= 95 (High); GL= 20 (High); Net carb= 21 g

Veal—Prime Rib: Breaded + fried ☛ Serving size= 3 oz, 85 g; GI= 95 (High); GL= 20 (High); Net carb= 21 g

Veal—Rib Steak Cuts: Breaded + fried ☛ Serving size= 3 oz, 85 g; GI= 95 (High); GL= 20 (High); Net carb= 21 g

Veal—Round Steak Varieties: Breaded + fried ☛ Serving size= 3 oz, 85 g; GI= 95 (High); GL= 20 (High); Net carb= 21 g

Veal—Short Loin: Breaded + fried ☛ Serving size= 3 oz, 85 g; GI= 95 (High); GL= 20 (High); Net carb= 21 g

Veal—Short Ribs: Breaded + fried ☛ Serving size= 3 oz, 85 g; GI= 95 (High); GL= 20 (High); Net carb= 21 g

Veal—T-Bone Steak: Breaded + fried ☛ Serving size= 3 oz, 85 g; GI= 95 (High); GL= 20 (High); Net carb= 21 g

Veal—Tenderloin: Breaded + fried ☛ Serving size= 3 oz, 85 g; GI= 95 (High); GL= 20 (High); Net carb= 21 g

Veal—Tongue: Breaded + fried ☛ Serving size= 1 slice, 81 g; GI= 95 (High); GL= 20 (High); Net carb= 21 g

Veal—Top Sirloin: Breaded + fried ☛ Serving size= 3 oz, 85 g; GI= 95 (High); GL= 20 (High); Net carb= 21 g

Veal—Tri-Tip: Breaded + fried ☛ Serving size= 3 oz, 85 g; GI= 95 (High); GL= 20 (High); Net carb= 21 g

Veal—Tripe: Breaded + fried ☛ Serving size= 3 oz, 85 g; GI= 95 (High); GL= 20 (High); Net carb= 21 g

39

BEVERAGES

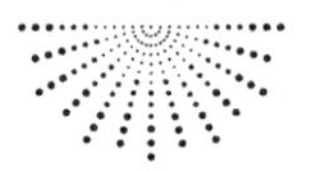

— People with diabetes should avoid heavy drinking

Alcoholic Beverage—Malt Beer Hard Lemonade ☛ Serving size= fl oz, 335 g; GI= 100 (High); GL= 33.7 (High); Net carb= 33.7 g

Carob-Flavor Beverage—Mix Powder Made With Whole Milk ☛ Serving size= 1 cup (8 fl oz), 256 g; GI= 100 (High); GL= 21.2 (High); Net carb= 21.2 g

Chocolate Syrup Made With Whole Milk ☛ Serving size= 1 cup (8 fl oz), 282 g; GI= 57 (Medium); GL= 20.1 (High); Net carb= 35.2 g

Chocolate-Flavor Beverage—Mix For Milk Powder With Added Nutrients Made With Whole Milk ☛ Serving size= 1 serving, 266 g; GI= 77 (High); GL= 23.5 (High); Net carb= 30.5 g

Chocolate-Flavor Beverage—Mix Powder Made With Whole Milk ☛ Serving size= 1 cup (8 fl oz), 266 g; GI= 77 (High); GL= 23.7 (High); Net carb= 30.7 g

Cocktail Mix Non-Alcoholic Concentrated Frozen ☛ Serving size= 1 fl oz, 36 g; GI= 79 (High); GL= 20.4 (High); Net carb= 25.8 g

Cranberry Juice Cocktail ☛ Serving size= 1 cup, 271 g; GI= 59 (Medium); GL= 19.6 (High); Net carb= 33.2 g

Energy Drink ☛ Serving size= 8 fl oz, 240 g; GI= 68 (Medium); GL= 24.5 (High); Net carb= 36 g

Energy Drink Full Throttle ☛ Serving size= 1 serving 8 fluid oz, 240 g; GI= 68 (Medium); GL= 19.7 (High); Net carb= 29 g

Energy Drink—Amp ☛ Serving size= 1 serving, 240 g; GI= 68 (Medium); GL= 19.7 (High); Net carb= 29 g

Fruit Flavored Drink Less Than 3% Juice Not Enriched With Vitamin C ☛ Serving size= 1 cup (8 fl oz), 238 g; GI= 68 (Medium); GL= 25.9 (High); Net carb= 38.2 g

Fruit Juice Drink—Greater Than 3% Fruit Juice High Vitamin C And Added Thiamin ☛ Serving size= 8 fl oz, 237 g; GI= 68 (Medium); GL= 21 (High); Net carb= 31 g

Horchata Beverage—Made With Milk ☛ Serving size= 1 cup, 248 g; GI= 45 (Low); GL= 21.5 (High); Net carb= 47.9 g

Horchata Beverage—Made With Water ☛ Serving size= 1 cup, 248 g; GI= 45 (Low); GL= 22.3 (High); Net carb= 49.6 g

Kiwi Strawberry Juice Drink ☛ Serving size= 16 fl oz, 473 g; GI= 68 (Medium); GL= 39.4 (High); Net carb= 58 g

Lemonada Limeade (Minute Maid) ☛ Serving size= 8 fl oz, 240 g; GI= 68 (Medium); GL= 22.4 (High); Net carb= 33 g

Lemonade (Minute Maid) ☛ Serving size= 8 fl oz, 240 g; GI= 68 (Medium); GL= 19.7 (High); Net carb= 29 g

Oatmeal Beverage—With Milk ☛ Serving size= 1 cup, 248 g; GI= 59 (Medium); GL= 22.5 (High); Net carb= 38.2 g

Orange Juice Drink ☛ Serving size= 1 cup, 249 g; GI= 68 (Medium); GL= 22.4 (High); Net carb= 32.9 g

Strawberry-Flavor Beverage—Mix Powder ☛ Serving size= 1 serving (2-3 heaping tsp), 22 g; GI= 89 (High); GL= 19.4 (High); Net carb= 21.8 g

Strawberry-Flavor Beverage—Mix Powder Made With Whole Milk ☛ Serving size= 1 cup (8 fl oz), 266 g; GI= 68 (Medium); GL= 22.2 (High); Net carb= 32.7 g

Tea—Black—Ready-To-Drink—Lemon Sweetened ☛ Serving size= 1 cup, 271 g; GI= 68 (Medium); GL= 19.9 (High); Net carb= 29.3 g

40

DAIRY AND SOY ALTERNATIVES

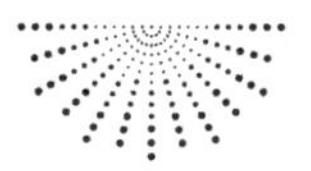

Milk shake—with malt ☛ Serving size: 1 cup (226g grams); GI= 53 (Low); GL= 21.6 (High); Net carb= 40.8 g

Milk shake—with malt ☛ Serving size: 1 cup (226g grams); GI= 53 (Low); GL= 21.6 (High); Net carb= 40.8 g

Milk—condensed, diluted, sweetened ☛ Serving size: 1 oz; GI= 61 (Medium); GL= 11.2 (High); Net carb= 18.4 g

Milk—condensed, sweetened, average value ☛ Serving size: 1 oz; GI= 61 (Medium); GL= 11.2 (High); Net carb= 18.4 g

Milk—condensed, undiluted, sweetened ☛ Serving size: 1 oz; GI= 61 (Medium); GL= 11.2 (High); Net carb= 18.4 g

41
LEGUMS AND BEANS

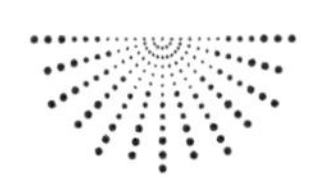

Beans Adzuki—Mature Seeds Canned Sweetened ☛ Serving size= ½ cup, 150 g; GI= 77 (High); GL= 63.5 (High); Net carb= 82.5 g

Beans Adzuki—Mature Seeds Raw ☛ Serving size= ½ cup, 150 g; GI= 33 (Low); GL= 24.8 (High); Net carb= 75.3 g

Black Beans—Turtle Mature Seeds Raw ☛ Serving size= ½ cup, 150 g; GI= 41 (Low); GL= 29.4 (High); Net carb= 71.6 g

Broad beans (Fava)—Mature Seeds Raw ☛ Serving size= ½ cup, 150 g; GI= 40 (Low); GL= 20 (High); Net carb= 49.9 g

Chickpeas (Garbanzo)—Mature Seeds Raw ☛ Serving size= ½ cup, 150 g; GI= 36 (Low); GL= 27.4 (High); Net carb= 76.1 g

Cowpeas—Mature Seeds Raw ☛ Serving size= ½ cup, 150 g; GI= 50 (Low); GL= 37.1 (High); Net carb= 74.1 g

Green Peas—Split Mature Seeds Raw ☛ Serving size= ½ cup, 150 g; GI= 51 (Low); GL= 30.2 (High); Net carb= 59.1 g

Hyacinth Beans—Mature Seeds Raw ☛ Serving size= ½ cup, 150 g; GI= 49 (Low); GL= 25.8 (High); Net carb= 52.7 g

Kidney Beans—All Types Mature Seeds Raw ☛ Serving size= ½ cup, 150 g; GI= 37 (Low); GL= 19.5 (High); Net carb= 52.7 g

Kidney Beans—Red Mature Seeds Raw ☛ Serving size= ½ cup, 150 g; GI= 37 (Low); GL= 25.6 (High); Net carb= 69.1 g

Lima Beans—Large Mature Seeds Raw ☛ Serving size= ½ cup, 150 g; GI= 46 (Low); GL= 30.6 (High); Net carb= 66.6 g

Mothbeans—Mature Seeds Raw ☛ Serving size= ½ cup, 150 g; GI= 51 (Low); GL= 47.1 (High); Net carb= 92.3 g

Mung Beans—Mature Seeds Raw ☛ Serving size= ½ cup, 150 g; GI= 42 (Low); GL= 29.2 (High); Net carb= 69.5 g

Navy Beans—Mature Seeds Raw ☛ Serving size= ½ cup, 150 g; GI= 39 (Low); GL= 26.6 (High); Net carb= 68.2 g

Pigeon Peas—Mature Seeds Raw ☛ Serving size= ½ cup, 150 g; GI= 31 (Low); GL= 22.2 (High); Net carb= 71.7 g

Pink Beans—Mature Seeds Raw ☛ Serving size= ½ cup, 150 g; GI= 37 (Low); GL= 28.6 (High); Net carb= 77.2 g

Pinto Beans—Mature Seeds Raw ☛ Serving size= ½ cup, 150 g; GI= 39 (Low); GL= 27.5 (High); Net carb= 70.6 g

Small White Beans—Mature Seeds Raw ☛ Serving size= ½ cup, 150 g; GI= 36 (Low); GL= 20.2 (High); Net carb= 56 g

Tofu Yogurt ☛ Serving size= 1 cup, 262 g; GI= 50 (Low); GL= 20.6 (High); Net carb= 41.3 g

White Beans—Mature Seeds Raw ☛ Serving size= ½ cup, 150 g; GI= 36 (Low); GL= 24.3 (High); Net carb= 67.6 g

Yardlong Beans—Mature Seeds Raw ☛ Serving size= 1 cup, 167 g; GI= 43 (Low); GL= 36.6 (High); Net carb= 85 g

Yellow Beans—Mature Seeds Raw ☛ Serving size= ½ cup, 150 g; GI= 36 (Low); GL= 19.2 (High); Net carb= 53.4 g

42
FISH & FISH PRODUCTS

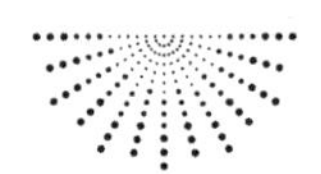

Fish stick—patty, or fillet ☛ Serving size= 3 0z (85 g); GI= 95 (High); GL= 37 (High)

Fish stick—patty, or fillet, baked or broiled ☛ Serving size= 3 0z (85 g); GI= 95 (High); GL= 37 (High)

Fish stick—patty, or fillet, battered, fried ☛ Serving size= 3 0z (85 g); GI= 95 (High); GL= 37 (High)

Fish stick—patty, or fillet, breaded or battered, baked ☛ Serving size= 3 0z (85 g); GI= 95 (High); GL= 37 (High)

43
FRUITS AND FRUITS PRODUCTS

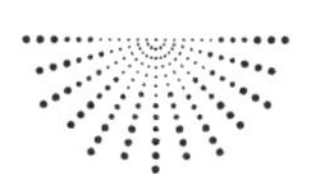

Apple Candied ☛ Serving size= 1 small apple, 198 (g); GI= 44 (Low); GL= 23.3 (High); Net carbs= 53 g

Apple Dried Cooked Without Sugar ☛ Serving size= 1 cup, 280 (g); GI= 45 (Low); GL= 28.5 (High); Net carbs= 63.3 g

Apples—Canned—sweetened Sliced Drained Heated ☛ Serving size= 1 cup slices, 204 (g); GI= 89 (High); GL= 26.9 (High); Net carbs= 30.3 g

Applesauce— Canned—sweetened, With Salt ☛ Serving size= 1 cup, 255 (g); GI= 89 (High); GL= 42.5 (High); Net carbs= 47.7 g

Applesauce—Canned—sweetened, Without Salt (Includes USDA Commodity) ☛ Serving size= 1 cup, 246 (g); GI= 77 (High); GL= 30.9 (High); Net carbs= 40.1 g

Apricot Dried Cooked, Without Sugar ☛ Serving size= 1 cup, nfs, 270 (g); GI= 41 (Low); GL= 31.2 (High); Net carbs= 76.1 g

Apricots—Dehydrated (Low-Moisture) Sulfured Stewed ☛ Serving size= 1 cup, 249 (g); GI= 31 (Low); GL= 25.2 (High); Net carbs= 81.2 g

Apricots—Frozen—sweetened ☛ Serving size= 1 cup, 242 (g); GI= 77 (High); GL= 42.7 (High); Net carbs= 55.4 g

Banana—Baked ☛ Serving size= 1 banana (7-1/4" long), 128 (g); GI= 53 (Low); GL= 20.1 (High); Net carbs= 38 g

Banana—Batter-Dipped Fried ☛ Serving size= 1 small, 108 (g); GI= 53 (Low); GL= 21.3 (High); Net carbs= 40.1 g

Banana—unripe ☛ Serving size= 1 cup, mashed, 225 (g); GI= 45 (Low); GL= 20.5 (High); Net carbs= 45.5 g

Blueberries—Canned—Heavy Syrup—Solids And Liquids ☛ Serving size= 1 cup, 256 (g); GI= 53 (Low); GL= 27.8 (High); Net carbs= 52.4 g

Blueberries—Canned Light Syrup Drained ☛ Serving size= 1 cup, 244 (g); GI= 53 (Low); GL= 25.9 (High); Net carbs= 48.9 g

Blueberries Frozen—sweetened ☛ Serving size= 1 cup, thawed, 230 (g); GI= 77 (High); GL= 35 (High); Net carbs= 45.4 g

Blueberries Wild—Canned Heavy Syrup Drained ☛ Serving size= 1 cup, 319 (g); GI= 53 (Low); GL= 39.6 (High); Net carbs= 74.7 g

Boysenberries—Canned Heavy Syrup ☛ Serving size= 1 cup, 256 (g); GI= 43 (Low); GL= 21.7 (High); Net carbs= 50.5 g

Breadfruit ☛ Serving size= 1 cup, 220 (g); GI= 65 (Medium); GL= 31.8 (High); Net carbs= 48.9 g

Cherries Sour Red—Canned—Extra Heavy Syrup Pack—Solids And Liquids ☛ Serving size= 1 cup, 261 (g); GI= 73 (High); GL= 54.2 (High); Net carbs= 74.2 g

Cherries Sour Red—Canned—Heavy Syrup Pack—Solids And Liquids ☛ Serving size= 1 cup, 256 (g); GI= 73 (High); GL= 41.4 (High); Net carbs= 56.8 g

Cherries Sour Red—Canned—Light Syrup Pack—Solids And Liquids ☛ Serving size= 1 cup, 252 (g); GI= 73 (High); GL= 34 (High); Net carbs= 46.6 g

Cherries Sweet—Canned—Extra Heavy Syrup Pack—Solids And Liquids ☛ Serving size= 1 cup, pitted, 261 (g); GI= 73 (High); GL= 47.1 (High); Net carbs= 64.5 g

Cherries Sweet—Canned—Juice—Pack—Solids And Liquids ☛ Serving size= 1 cup, pitted, 250 (g); GI= 73 (High); GL= 22.5 (High); Net carbs= 30.8 g

Cherries Sweet—Canned—Light Syrup Pack—Solids And Liquids ☛ Serving size= 1 cup, pitted, 252 (g); GI= 73 (High); GL= 29 (High); Net carbs= 39.8 g

Cherries Sweet—Canned Pitted Heavy Syrup Drained ☛ Serving size= 1 cup, 179 (g); GI= 73 (High); GL= 24.5 (High); Net carbs= 33.6 g

Cherries Sweet—Canned—Pitted Heavy Syrup Pack—Solids And Liquids ☛ Serving size= 1 cup, 253 (g); GI= 73 (High); GL= 36.7 (High); Net carbs= 50.3 g

Cherries Tart Dried—sweetened ☛ Serving size= 1/4 cup, 40 (g); GI= 87 (High); GL= 27.1 (High); Net carbs= 31.2 g

Cranberry Sauce—Canned—sweetened ☛ Serving size= 1 cup, 277 (g); GI= 77 (High); GL= 83.8 (High); Net carbs= 108.9 g

Cranberry-Orange Relish—Canned ☛ Serving size= 1 cup, 275 (g); GI= 77 (High); GL= 97.8 (High); Net carbs= 127.1 g

Dried Apples ☛ Serving size= 1 cup, 86 (g); GI= 45 (Low); GL= 22.1 (High); Net carbs= 49.2 g

Dried Apricots ☛ Serving size= 1 cup, halves, 130 (g); GI= 41 (Low); GL= 29.5 (High); Net carbs= 71.9 g

Dried Bananas ☛ Serving size= 1 cup, 100 (g); GI= 63 (Medium); GL= 49.4 (High); Net carbs= 78.4 g

Dried Blueberries (Sweetened) ☛ Serving size= 1/4 cup, 40 (g); GI= 73 (High); GL= 21.2 (High); Net carbs= 29 g

Dried Cranberries (Sweetened) ☛ Serving size= 1/4 cup, 40 (g); GI= 73 (High); GL= 22.6 (High); Net carbs= 31 g

Dried Figs ☛ Serving size= 1 cup, 149 (g); GI= 61 (Medium); GL= 49.1 (High); Net carbs= 80.6 g

Dried Peaches ☛ Serving size= 1 cup, halves, 160 (g); GI= 52 (Low); GL= 44.2 (High); Net carbs= 85 g

Dried Pears ☛ Serving size= 1 cup, halves, 180 (g); GI= 54 (Low); GL= 60.5 (High); Net carbs= 112 g

Durian ☛ Serving size= 1 cup, chopped or diced, 243 (g); GI= 49 (Low); GL= 27.7 (High); Net carbs= 56.6 g

Fig Dried Cooked With Sugar ☛ Serving size= 1 cup, 270 (g); GI= 83 (High); GL= 70.7 (High); Net carbs= 85.1 g

Figs—Canned—Extra Heavy Syrup Pack—Solids And Liquids ☛ Serving size= 1 cup, 261 (g); GI= 82 (High); GL= 59.6 (High); Net carbs= 72.7 g

Figs—Canned—Heavy Syrup Pack—Solids And Liquids ☛ Serving size= 1 cup, 259 (g); GI= 82 (High); GL= 44 (High); Net carbs= 53.6 g

Figs—Canned—Light Syrup Pack—Solids And Liquids ☛ Serving size= 1 cup, 252 (g); GI= 82 (High); GL= 33.4 (High); Net carbs= 40.7 g

Figs—Canned—Water Pack—Solids And Liquids ☛ Serving size= 1 cup, 248 (g); GI= 82 (High); GL= 24 (High); Net carbs= 29.2 g

Figs Dried Stewed ☛ Serving size= 1 cup, 259 (g); GI= 61 (Medium); GL= 36.9 (High); Net carbs= 60.5 g

Fruit Cocktail—(Peach And Pineapple And Pear And Grape And Cherry)—Canned—Extra Heavy Syrup—Solids And Liquids ☛ Serving size= 1/2 cup, 130 (g); GI= 79 (High); GL= 22.4 (High); Net carbs= 28.3 g

Fruit Cocktail—(Peach And Pineapple And Pear And Grape And

Cherry)—Canned—Heavy Syrup—Solids And Liquids ☛ Serving size= 1 cup, 248 (g); GI= 79 (High); GL= 35.1 (High); Net carbs= 44.4 g

Fruit Cocktail—(Peach And Pineapple And Pear And Grape And Cherry)—Canned—Juice Pack—Solids And Liquids ☛ Serving size= 1 cup, 237 (g); GI= 79 (High); GL= 20.3 (High); Net carbs= 25.7 g

Fruit Cocktail—(Peach And Pineapple And Pear And Grape And Cherry)—Canned—Light Syrup—Solids And Liquids ☛ Serving size= 1 cup, 242 (g); GI= 79 (High); GL= 26.6 (High); Net carbs= 33.7 g

Fruit Cocktail—Canned Heavy Syrup Drained ☛ Serving size= 1 cup, 214 (g); GI= 79 (High); GL= 28.9 (High); Net carbs= 36.6 g

Fruit Juice—Smoothie—Naked Juice—Mighty Mango ☛ Serving size= 8 fl oz, 240 (g); GI= 77 (High); GL= 27.7 (High); Net carbs= 36 g

Fruit Juice—Smoothie—Naked Juice—Strawberry Banana ☛ Serving size= 1 cup, 228 (g); GI= 76 (High); GL= 19.2 (High); Net carbs= 25.2 g

Fruit Salad—(Peach And Pear And Apricot And Pineapple And Cherry)—Canned—Extra Heavy Syrup—Solids And Liquids ☛ Serving size= 1 cup, 259 (g); GI= 68 (Medium); GL= 38.3 (High); Net carbs= 56.4 g

Fruit Salad—(Peach And Pear And Apricot And Pineapple And Cherry)—Canned—Light Syrup—Solids And Liquids ☛ Serving size= 1 cup, 252 (g); GI= 68 (Medium); GL= 24.2 (High); Net carbs= 35.6 g

Fruit Salad—(Pineapple And Papaya And Banana And Guava) Tropical —Canned—Heavy Syrup—Solids And Liquids ☛ Serving size= 1 cup, 257 (g); GI= 68 (Medium); GL= 36.8 (High); Net carbs= 54.1 g

Golden Seedless Raisins ☛ Serving size= 1 cup, packed, 165 (g); GI= 53 (Low); GL= 67.1 (High); Net carbs= 126.6 g

Gooseberries—Canned—Light Syrup Pack—Solids And Liquids ☛

Serving size= 1 cup, 252 (g); GI= 78 (High); GL= 32.1 (High); Net carbs= 41.2 g

Grape Juice ☛ Serving size= 1 cup, 253 (g); GI= 66 (Medium); GL= 24.3 (High); Net carbs= 36.9 g

Grapefruit And Orange Sections Cooked—Canned Or Frozen In Light Syrup ☛ Serving size= 1 cup, 254 (g); GI= 75 (High); GL= 27.3 (High); Net carbs= 36.4 g

Grapefruit—Juice—White—Canned—sweetened ☛ Serving size= 1 cup, 250 (g); GI= 77 (High); GL= 21.2 (High); Net carbs= 27.6 g

Grapefruit—Juice—White Frozen Concentrate—unsweetened Undiluted ☛ Serving size= 1 can (6 fl oz), 207 (g); GI= 59 (Medium); GL= 41.7 (High); Net carbs= 70.7 g

Grapefruit Sections—Canned—Light Syrup Pack—Solids And Liquids ☛ Serving size= 1 cup, 254 (g); GI= 77 (High); GL= 29.4 (High); Net carbs= 38.2 g

Grapes—Canned—Thompson Seedless Heavy Syrup Pack—Solids And Liquids ☛ Serving size= 1 cup, 256 (g); GI= 77 (High); GL= 37.6 (High); Net carbs= 48.8 g

Guanabana Nectar—Canned ☛ Serving size= 1 cup, 251 (g); GI= 63 (Medium); GL= 23.5 (High); Net carbs= 37.2 g

Guava Nectar With Sucralose—Canned ☛ Serving size= fl oz, 335 (g); GI= 61 (Medium); GL= 24.7 (High); Net carbs= 40.5 g

Guava Shell—Canned In Heavy Syrup ☛ Serving size= 1 cup, 310 (g); GI= 61 (Medium); GL= 41.7 (High); Net carbs= 68.3 g

Jackfruit—Canned Syrup Pack ☛ Serving size= 1 cup, drained, 178 (g); GI= 81 (High); GL= 33.2 (High); Net carbs= 41 g

Mango Nectar—Canned ☛ Serving size= 1 cup, 251 (g); GI= 69 (Medium); GL= 22.2 (High); Net carbs= 32.2 g

Mangosteen—Canned Syrup Pack ☛ Serving size= 1 cup, drained, 196 (g); GI= 67 (Medium); GL= 21.2 (High); Net carbs= 31.6 g

Orange Juice—Frozen Concentrate—unsweetened Undiluted ☛ Serving size= 1 cup, 262 (g); GI= 59 (Medium); GL= 52.9 (High); Net carbs= 89.6 g

Orange Pineapple Juice—Blend ☛ Serving size= 8 fl oz, 246 (g); GI= 66 (Medium); GL= 19.5 (High); Net carbs= 29.5 g

Papaya Cooked Or Canned In Sugar Or Syrup ☛ Serving size= 1 cup, 244 (g); GI= 72 (High); GL= 33.6 (High); Net carbs= 46.7 g

Papaya Nectar—Canned ☛ Serving size= 1 cup, 250 (g); GI= 72 (High); GL= 25 (High); Net carbs= 34.8 g

Peach Dried Cooked With Sugar ☛ Serving size= 1 cup, 270 (g); GI= 83 (High); GL= 58 (High); Net carbs= 69.9 g

Peaches—Canned—Extra Heavy Syrup Pack—Solids And Liquids ☛ Serving size= 1 cup, halves or slices, 262 (g); GI= 81 (High); GL= 53.2 (High); Net carbs= 65.7 g

Peaches—Canned—Extra Light Syrup—Solids And Liquids ☛ Serving size= 1 cup, halves or slices, 247 (g); GI= 81 (High); GL= 20.2 (High); Net carbs= 24.9 g

Peaches—Canned Heavy Syrup Drained ☛ Serving size= 1 cup, 222 (g); GI= 81 (High); GL= 31 (High); Net carbs= 38.3 g

Peaches—Canned—Heavy Syrup Pack—Solids And Liquids ☛ Serving size= 1 cup, 262 (g); GI= 81 (High); GL= 39.6 (High); Net carbs= 48.8 g

Peaches—Canned—Juice—Pack—Solids And Liquids ☛ Serving size= 1 cup, 250 (g); GI= 81 (High); GL= 20.8 (High); Net carbs= 25.7 g

Peaches—Canned—Light Syrup Pack—Solids And Liquids ☛ Serving size= 1 cup, halves or slices, 251 (g); GI= 81 (High); GL= 26.9 (High); Net carbs= 33.3 g

Peaches Dehydrated (Low-Moisture) Sulfured Stewed ☛ Serving size= 1 cup, 242 (g); GI= 50 (Low); GL= 41.3 (High); Net carbs= 82.6 g

Peaches Frozen Sliced—sweetened ☛ Serving size= 1 cup, thawed, 250 (g); GI= 77 (High); GL= 42.7 (High); Net carbs= 55.5 g

Peaches Spiced—Canned—Heavy Syrup Pack—Solids And Liquids ☛ Serving size= 1 cup, whole, 242 (g); GI= 83 (High); GL= 37.7 (High); Net carbs= 45.4 g

Pear Dried Cooked Without Sugar ☛ Serving size= 1 cup, 280 (g); GI= 52 (Low); GL= 51.3 (High); Net carbs= 98.6 g

Pears—Canned—Extra Light Syrup Pack—Solids And Liquids ☛ Serving size= 1 cup, halves, 247 (g); GI= 83 (High); GL= 21.7 (High); Net carbs= 26.2 g

Pears—Canned Heavy Syrup Drained ☛ Serving size= 1 cup, 201 (g); GI= 83 (High); GL= 27.3 (High); Net carbs= 32.9 g

Pears—Canned—Heavy Syrup Pack—Solids And Liquids ☛ Serving size= 1 cup, 266 (g); GI= 83 (High); GL= 38.8 (High); Net carbs= 46.7 g

Pears—Canned In Syrup ☛ Serving size= 1 cup, halves, 266 (g); GI= 83 (High); GL= 52.2 (High); Net carbs= 62.9 g

Pears—Canned—Juice—Pack—Solids And Liquids ☛ Serving size= 1 cup, halves, 248 (g); GI= 83 (High); GL= 23.3 (High); Net carbs= 28.1 g

Pears—Canned—Light Syrup Pack—Solids And Liquids ☛ Serving size= 1 cup, halves, 251 (g); GI= 83 (High); GL= 28.3 (High); Net carbs= 34.1 g

Pineapple—Canned—Extra Heavy Syrup Pack—Solids And Liquids ☛ Serving size= 1 cup, crushed, sliced, or chunks, 260 (g); GI= 79 (High); GL= 42.5 (High); Net carbs= 53.8 g

Pineapple—Canned—Heavy Syrup Pack—Solids And Liquids ☛

Serving size= 1 cup, crushed, sliced, or chunks, 254 (g); GI= 79 (High); GL= 38.9 (High); Net carbs= 49.3 g

Pineapple—Canned Juice—Pack Drained ☛ Serving size= 1 cup, chunks, 181 (g); GI= 79 (High); GL= 20.4 (High); Net carbs= 25.8 g

Pineapple—Canned—Juice—Pack—Solids And Liquids ☛ Serving size= 1 cup, crushed, sliced, or chunks, 249 (g); GI= 79 (High); GL= 29.3 (High); Net carbs= 37.1 g

Pineapple—Canned—Light Syrup Pack—Solids And Liquids ☛ Serving size= 1 cup, crushed, sliced, or chunks, 252 (g); GI= 79 (High); GL= 25.2 (High); Net carbs= 31.9 g

Pineapple Frozen Chunks—sweetened ☛ Serving size= 1 cup, chunks, 245 (g); GI= 77 (High); GL= 39.8 (High); Net carbs= 51.7 g

Pineapple Juice—Frozen Concentrate—unsweetened Diluted With 3 Volume Water ☛ Serving size= 1 cup, 250 (g); GI= 79 (High); GL= 24.6 (High); Net carbs= 31.2 g

Pineapple Juice—Frozen Concentrate—unsweetened Undiluted ☛ Serving size= 1 can (6 fl oz), 216 (g); GI= 79 (High); GL= 74.4 (High); Net carbs= 94.2 g

Plantains Cooked ☛ Serving size= 1 cup, mashed, 200 (g); GI= 40 (Low); GL= 31.3 (High); Net carbs= 78.3 g

Plantains Green Fried ☛ Serving size= 1 cup, 118 (g); GI= 40 (Low); GL= 21.6 (High); Net carbs= 53.9 g

Plums—Canned Heavy Syrup Drained ☛ Serving size= 1 cup, with pits, yields, 183 (g); GI= 78 (High); GL= 30.9 (High); Net carbs= 39.6 g

Plums—Canned—Purple Extra Heavy Syrup Pack—Solids And Liquids ☛ Serving size= 1 cup, pitted, 261 (g); GI= 78 (High); GL= 51.5 (High); Net carbs= 66.1 g

Plums—Canned—Purple Heavy Syrup Pack—Solids And Liquids ☛

Serving size= 1 cup, pitted, 258 (g); GI= 78 (High); GL= 45 (High); Net carbs= 57.6 g

Plums—Canned—Purple Juice—Pack—Solids And Liquids ☛ Serving size= 1 cup, pitted, 252 (g); GI= 78 (High); GL= 28 (High); Net carbs= 35.9 g

Plums—Canned—Purple Light Syrup Pack—Solids And Liquids ☛ Serving size= 1 cup, pitted, 252 (g); GI= 78 (High); GL= 30.2 (High); Net carbs= 38.8 g

Plums—Canned—Purple Water Pack—Solids And Liquids ☛ Serving size= 1 cup, pitted, 249 (g); GI= 78 (High); GL= 19.7 (High); Net carbs= 25.2 g

Pomegranate Juice—Bottled ☛ Serving size= 1 cup, 249 (g); GI= 67 (Medium); GL= 21.7 (High); Net carbs= 32.4 g

Prunes ☛ Serving size= 1 cup, 132 (g); GI= 29 (Low); GL= 34.1 (High); Net carbs= 117.6 g

Prunes—Canned—Heavy Syrup Pack—Solids And Liquids ☛ Serving size= 1 cup, 234 (g); GI= 78 (High); GL= 43.8 (High); Net carbs= 56.2 g

Prunes Dehydrated (Low-Moisture) Stewed ☛ Serving size= 1 cup, 280 (g); GI= 39 (Low); GL= 32.4 (High); Net carbs= 83.2 g

Raisins ☛ Serving size= 1 cup, packed, 165 (g); GI= 59 (Medium); GL= 72.8 (High); Net carbs= 123.5 g

Raisins Cooked ☛ Serving size= 1 cup, 295 (g); GI= 61 (Medium); GL= 100.2 (High); Net carbs= 164.3 g

Rambutan—Canned Syrup Pack ☛ Serving size= 1 cup, drained, 150 (g); GI= 77 (High); GL= 23.1 (High); Net carbs= 30 g

Raspberries—Canned—Red Heavy Syrup Pack—Solids And Liquids ☛ Serving size= 1 cup, 256 (g); GI= 77 (High); GL= 39.5 (High); Net carbs= 51.4 g

Raspberries Frozen Red—sweetened ☛ Serving size= 1 cup, thawed, 250 (g); GI= 77 (High); GL= 41.9 (High); Net carbs= 54.4 g

Rhubarb Cooked Or Canned Drained Solids ☛ Serving size= 1 cup, 240 (g); GI= 77 (High); GL= 54 (High); Net carbs= 70.1 g

Rhubarb Cooked Or Canned In Light Syrup ☛ Serving size= 1 cup, 240 (g); GI= 77 (High); GL= 25.3 (High); Net carbs= 32.8 g

Rhubarb Frozen Cooked With Sugar ☛ Serving size= 1 cup, 240 (g); GI= 77 (High); GL= 54 (High); Net carbs= 70.1 g

Shredded Coconut Meat (Sweetened) ☛ Serving size= 1 cup, 256 (g); GI= 77 (High); GL= 32.4 (High); Net carbs= 42.1 g

Starfruit Cooked With Sugar ☛ Serving size= 1 cup, 205 (g); GI= 77 (High); GL= 22.4 (High); Net carbs= 29.2 g

Strawberries—Canned—Heavy Syrup Pack—Solids And Liquids ☛ Serving size= 1 cup, 254 (g); GI= 75 (High); GL= 41.6 (High); Net carbs= 55.4 g

Strawberries Frozen—sweetened Sliced ☛ Serving size= 1 cup, thawed, 255 (g); GI= 75 (High); GL= 45.9 (High); Net carbs= 61.3 g

Tangerines (Mandarin Oranges)—Canned Light Syrup Pack ☛ Serving size= 1 cup, 252 (g); GI= 59 (Medium); GL= 23 (High); Net carbs= 39 g

44
GRAINS AND PASTA

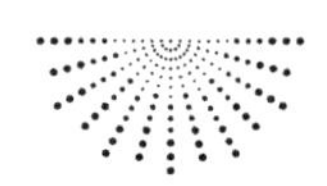

Amaranth Grain Uncooked ☛ Serving size= 1 cup (193 g); GI= 95 (High); GL= 107.4 (High); Net carb= 113 g

Barley—Flour Or Meal ☛ Serving size= 1 cup (148 g); GI= 31 (Low); GL= 29.6 (High); Net carb= 95.3 g

Barley—Hulled ☛ Serving size= 1 cup (184 g); GI= 25 (Low); GL= 25.8 (High); Net carb= 103.4 g

Barley—Malt Flour ☛ Serving size= 1 cup (162 g); GI= 40 (Low); GL= 46.1 (High); Net carb= 115.3 g

Barley—Pearled Raw ☛ Serving size= 1 cup (200 g); GI= 25 (Low); GL= 31.1 (High); Net carb= 124.2 g

Boiled Brown Rice ☛ Serving size= 1 cup (195 g); GI= 68 (Medium); GL= 28.8 (High); Net carb= 42.3 g

Brown Rice ☛ Serving size= 1 cup (202 g); GI= 68 (Medium); GL= 32.9 (High); Net carb= 48.4 g

Buckwheat (Uncooked) ☛ Serving size= 1 cup (170 g); GI= 55 (Medium); GL= 57.5 (High); Net carb= 104.6 g

Buckwheat Groats Roasted Dry ☛ Serving size= 1 cup (164 g); GI= 55 (Medium); GL= 58.3 (High); Net carb= 106 g

Bulgur Dry ☛ Serving size= 1 cup (140 g); GI= 47 (Low); GL= 41.7 (High); Net carb= 88.7 g

Cooked Amaranth ☛ Serving size= 1 cup (246 g); GI= 95 (High); GL= 38.8 (High); Net carb= 40.8 g

Cooked Couscous ☛ Serving size= 1 cup, cooked (157 g); GI= 65 (Medium); GL= 22.3 (High); Net carb= 34.3 g

Cooked Spelt ☛ Serving size= 1 cup (194 g); GI= 55 (Medium); GL= 24.1 (High); Net carb= 43.7 g

Corn Grain White ☛ Serving size= 1 cup (166 g); GI= 55 (Medium); GL= 67.8 (High); Net carb= 123.3 g

Corn Grain Yellow ☛ Serving size= 1 cup (166 g); GI= 59 (Medium); GL= 65.6 (High); Net carb= 111.2 g

Cornmeal—Degermed Unenriched White ☛ Serving size= 1 cup (157 g); GI= 68 (Medium); GL= 80.7 (High); Net carb= 118.6 g

Cornmeal—Degermed Unenriched Yellow ☛ Serving size= 1 cup (157 g); GI= 68 (Medium); GL= 80.7 (High); Net carb= 118.6 g

Cornmeal—Degermed, fortified White ☛ Serving size= 1 cup (157 g); GI= 68 (Medium); GL= 80.7 (High); Net carb= 118.6 g

Cornmeal—Degermed, fortified Yellow ☛ Serving size= 1 cup (157 g); GI= 68 (Medium); GL= 80.7 (High); Net carb= 118.6 g

Cornmeal—White Self-Rising Bolted With Wheat Flour Added, fortified ☛ Serving size= 1 cup (170 g); GI= 68 (Medium); GL= 77.6 (High); Net carb= 114.1 g

Cornmeal—White Self-Rising Degermed, fortified ☛ Serving size= 1 cup (138 g); GI= 68 (Medium); GL= 63.5 (High); Net carb= 93.4 g

Cornmeal—Yellow Self-Rising Bolted Plain, fortified ☛ Serving size= 1 cup (122 g); GI= 68 (Medium); GL= 52.7 (High); Net carb= 77.6 g

Cornmeal—Yellow Self-Rising Bolted With Wheat Flour Added, fortified ☛ Serving size= 1 cup (170 g); GI= 68 (Medium); GL= 77.6 (High); Net carb= 114.1 g

Cornmeal—Yellow Self-Rising Degermed, fortified ☛ Serving size= 1 cup (138 g); GI= 68 (Medium); GL= 63.5 (High); Net carb= 93.4 g

Cornstarch ☛ Serving size= 1 cup (128 g); GI= 97 (High); GL= 112.2 (High); Net carb= 115.7 g

Couscous Dry ☛ Serving size= 1 cup (173 g); GI= 65 (Medium); GL= 81.4 (High); Net carb= 125.3 g

Couscous Plain Cooked ☛ Serving size= 1 cup, cooked (160 g); GI= 65 (Medium); GL= 22.6 (High); Net carb= 34.7 g

Flour—Amaranth ☛ Serving size= 1 cup (137 g); GI= 105 (High); GL= 100.7 (High); Net carb= 95.9 g

Flour—Arrowroot ☛ Serving size= 1 cup (128 g); GI= 71 (High); GL= 77 (High); Net carb= 108.5 g

Flour—Barley ☛ Serving size= 1 cup (148 g); GI= 31 (Low); GL= 29.6 (High); Net carb= 95.3 g

Flour—Buckwheat Whole-Groat ☛ Serving size= 1 cup (120 g); GI= 70 (High); GL= 50.9 (High); Net carb= 72.7 g

Flour—Corn ☛ Serving size= 1 cup (137 g); GI= 87 (High); GL= 85.8 (High); Net carb= 98.6 g

Flour—Corn, Masa Unenriched White ☛ Serving size= 1 cup (114 g); GI= 87 (High); GL= 69.6 (High); Net carb= 80 g

Flour—Corn, Masa, fortified White ☛ Serving size= 1 cup (114 g); GI= 87 (High); GL= 69.6 (High); Net carb= 80 g

Flour—Corn, Whole-Grain White ☛ Serving size= 1 cup (117 g); GI= 87 (High); GL= 70.8 (High); Net carb= 81.4 g

Flour—Corn, Whole-Grain Yellow ☛ Serving size= 1 cup (117 g); GI= 87 (High); GL= 70.8 (High); Net carb= 81.4 g

Flour—Corn, yellow ☛ Serving size= 1 cup (137 g); GI= 87 (High); GL= 97 (High); Net carb= 111.5 g

Flour—Corn, Yellow Degermed Unenriched ☛ Serving size= 1 cup (126 g); GI= 87 (High); GL= 88.6 (High); Net carb= 101.9 g

Flour—Corn, Yellow Masa, fortified ☛ Serving size= 1 cup (114 g); GI= 87 (High); GL= 69.6 (High); Net carb= 80 g

Flour—Maize ☛ Serving size= 1 cup (137 g); GI= 94 (High); GL= 103 (High); Net carb= 109.6 g

Flour—Maize, starch ☛ Serving size= 1 cup (137 g); GI= 94 (High); GL= 103 (High); Net carb= 109.6 g

Flour—Oat, Partially Debranned ☛ Serving size= 1 cup (104 g); GI= 44 (Low); GL= 27.1 (High); Net carb= 61.6 g

Flour—Potato, starch ☛ Serving size= 1 cup (137 g); GI= 85 (High); GL= 97.8 (High); Net carb= 115.1 g

Flour—Rice Brown ☛ Serving size= 1 cup (158 g); GI= 63 (Medium); GL= 71.5 (High); Net carb= 113.6 g

Flour—Rye, Dark ☛ Serving size= 1 cup (128 g); GI= 57 (Medium); GL= 32.7 (High); Net carb= 57.4 g

Flour—Rye, Light ☛ Serving size= 1 cup (102 g); GI= 62 (Medium); GL= 43.4 (High); Net carb= 70.1 g

Flour—Rye, Medium ☛ Serving size= 1 cup (102 g); GI= 62 (Medium); GL= 40.2 (High); Net carb= 64.9 g

Flour—White Wheat ☛ Serving size= 1 cup (137 g); GI= 85 (High); GL= 85.7 (High); Net carb= 100.8 g

Flour—White Wheat, Bread, fortified ☛ Serving size= 1 cup (137 g); GI= 85 (High); GL= 81.7 (High); Net carb= 96.1 g

Flour—White Wheat, fortified Bleached ☛ Serving size= 1 cup (125 g); GI= 85 (High); GL= 78.2 (High); Net carb= 92 g

Flour—White Wheat, Self-Rising, fortified ☛ Serving size= 1 cup (125 g); GI= 85 (High); GL= 76 (High); Net carb= 89.4 g

Flour—White Wheat, Unenriched ☛ Serving size= 1 cup (125 g); GI= 85 (High); GL= 78.2 (High); Net carb= 92 g

Flour—White Wheat,, fortified Calcium-Fortified ☛ Serving size= 1 cup (125 g); GI= 85 (High); GL= 78.2 (High); Net carb= 92 g

Flour—White Wheat,, fortified Unbleached ☛ Serving size= 1 cup (125 g); GI= 85 (High); GL= 78.2 (High); Net carb= 92 g

Macaroni Vegetable, fortified Dry ☛ Serving size= 1 cup spiral shaped (84 g); GI= 50 (Low); GL= 29.6 (High); Net carb= 59.3 g

Medium Grain White Rice ☛ Serving size= 1 cup (186 g); GI= 68 (Medium); GL= 35.8 (High); Net carb= 52.6 g

Millet Flour ☛ Serving size= 1 cup (119 g); GI= 53 (Low); GL= 45.2 (High); Net carb= 85.2 g

Millet Raw ☛ Serving size= 1 cup (200 g); GI= 53 (Low); GL= 68.2 (High); Net carb= 128.7 g

Millet—(cooked with added fat) ☛ Serving size= 1 cup, cooked (170 g); GI= 53 (Low); GL= 19.1 (High); Net carb= 36 g

Millet—Finger millet ☛ Serving size= 1 cup (174 g); GI= 104 (High); GL= 129.1 (High); Net carb= 124.1 g

Millet—Foxtail millet ☛ Serving size= 1 cup (174 g); GI= 59 (Medium); GL= 73.2 (High); Net carb= 124.1 g

Millet—Kodo millet ☛ Serving size= 1 cup (174 g); GI= 65 (Medium); GL= 80.7 (High); Net carb= 124.1 g

Millet—Little millet ☛ Serving size= 1 cup (174 g); GI= 52 (Low); GL= 64.5 (High); Net carb= 124.1 g

Millet—Pearl millet ☛ Serving size= 1 cup (174 g); GI= 54 (Low); GL= 50.7 (High); Net carb= 94 g

Noodles—Cooked ☛ Serving size= 1 cup, cooked (160 g); GI= 55 (Medium); GL= 21 (High); Net carb= 38.1 g

Noodles—Egg (Cooked) ☛ Serving size= 1 cup (160 g); GI= 55 (Medium); GL= 21.1 (High); Net carb= 38.3 g

Noodles—Egg Cooked Unfortified With Added Salt ☛ Serving size= 1 cup (160 g); GI= 55 (Medium); GL= 21.1 (High); Net carb= 38.3 g

Noodles—Egg Cooked, fortified With Added Salt ☛ Serving size= 1 cup (160 g); GI= 55 (Medium); GL= 21.1 (High); Net carb= 38.3 g

Noodles—Egg Unfortified, Cooked Without Added Salt ☛ Serving size= 1 cup (160 g); GI= 55 (Medium); GL= 21.1 (High); Net carb= 38.3 g

Noodles—Japanese Somen Dry ☛ Serving size= 1 cup (176 g); GI= 41 (Low); GL= 50.4 (High); Net carb= 122.8 g

Noodles—Long Rice, prepared from Mung Beans Cooked ☛ Serving size= 1 cup, cooked (190 g); GI= 55 (Medium); GL= 21.5 (High); Net carb= 39.1 g

Noodles—Rice Dry ☛ Serving size= 2 oz (57 g); GI= 56 (Medium); GL= 25.1 (High); Net carb= 44.8 g

Noodles—Whole Grain Cooked ☛ Serving size= 1 cup, cooked (160 g); GI= 53 (Low); GL= 22.1 (High); Net carb= 41.6 g

Oat Bran ☛ Serving size= 1 cup (94 g); GI= 77 (High); GL= 36.8 (High); Net carb= 47.8 g

Pasta—Brown Rice Flour, Gluten-Free, Cooked Tinkyada ☛ Serving size= 1 cup spaghetti not packed (169 g); GI= 71 (High); GL= 36.6 (High); Net carb= 51.5 g

Pasta—Cooked ☛ Serving size= 1 cup, cooked (140 g); GI= 63 (Medium); GL= 25.5 (High); Net carb= 40.4 g

Pasta—Cooked Unenriched With Added Salt ☛ Serving size= 1 cup spaghetti not packed (124 g); GI= 63 (Medium); GL= 22.5 (High); Net carb= 35.7 g

Pasta—Cooked, fortified With Added Salt ☛ Serving size= 1 cup spaghetti not packed (124 g); GI= 63 (Medium); GL= 22.5 (High); Net carb= 35.7 g

Pasta—Cooked, fortified Without Added Salt ☛ Serving size= 1 cup spaghetti not packed (124 g); GI= 63 (Medium); GL= 22.7 (High); Net carb= 36 g

Pasta—Corn And Rice Flour, Gluten-Free, Cooked ☛ Serving size= 1 cup spaghetti (141 g); GI= 71 (High); GL= 36.7 (High); Net carb= 51.7 g

Pasta—Corn Flour And Quinoa Flour, Gluten-Free, Cooked Ancient Harvest ☛ Serving size= 1 cup spaghetti packed (166 g); GI= 70 (High); GL= 32.3 (High); Net carb= 46.2 g

Pasta—Corn, Gluten-Free, Dry ☛ Serving size= 1 cup (105 g); GI= 78 (High); GL= 55.9 (High); Net carb= 71.7 g

Pasta—Dry Unenriched ☛ Serving size= 1 cup spaghetti (91 g); GI= 63 (Medium); GL= 41 (High); Net carb= 65 g

Pasta—Dry, fortified ☛ Serving size= 1 cup spaghetti (91 g); GI= 63 (Medium); GL= 41 (High); Net carb= 65 g

Pasta—Fresh-Refrigerated Plain As Purchased ☛ Serving size= 4 (1/2) oz (128 g); GI= 58 (Medium); GL= 40.6 (High); Net carb= 70.1 g

Pasta—Fresh-Refrigerated Spinach As Purchased ☛ Serving size= 4 (1/2) oz (128 g); GI= 58 (Medium); GL= 41.4 (High); Net carb= 71.3 g

Pasta—Gluten-Free Rice Flour And Rice Bran Extract Cooked De

Boles ☛ Serving size= 1 cup spaghetti (121 g); GI= 63 (Medium); GL= 29.6 (High); Net carb= 47 g

Pasta—Whole Grain Cooked ☛ Serving size= 1 cup, cooked (140 g); GI= 61 (Medium); GL= 22.2 (High); Net carb= 36.4 g

Quinoa—Cooked ☛ Serving size= 1 cup (185 g); GI= 50 (Low); GL= 26.4 (High); Net carb= 52.7 g

Quinoa—Uncooked ☛ Serving size= 1 cup (170 g); GI= 53 (Low); GL= 51.5 (High); Net carb= 97.2 g

Rice Brown And Wild—Cooked (cooked without added fat) ☛ Serving size= 1 cup, cooked (151 g); GI= 56 (Medium); GL= 19.7 (High); Net carb= 35.2 g

Rice Brown—Cooked (cooked with added fat) Made With Oil ☛ Serving size= 1 cup, cooked (196 g); GI= 56 (Medium); GL= 25.5 (High); Net carb= 45.6 g

Rice Brown—Cooked (cooked without added fat) ☛ Serving size= 1 cup, cooked (196 g); GI= 56 (Medium); GL= 26.2 (High); Net carb= 46.7 g

Rice Brown—Long-Grain Raw ☛ Serving size= 1 cup (185 g); GI= 51 (Low); GL= 68.5 (High); Net carb= 134.4 g

Rice Brown—Medium-Grain Raw ☛ Serving size= 1 cup (190 g); GI= 56 (Medium); GL= 77.4 (High); Net carb= 138.3 g

Rice White And Wild—Cooked (cooked with added fat) ☛ Serving size= 1 cup, cooked (151 g); GI= 72 (High); GL= 21.9 (High); Net carb= 30.4 g

Rice White And Wild—Cooked (cooked without added fat) ☛ Serving size= 1 cup, cooked (164 g); GI= 72 (High); GL= 30 (High); Net carb= 41.6 g

Rice White—Cooked (cooked with added fat) Made With Oil ☛

Serving size= 1 cup, cooked (163 g); GI= 72 (High); GL= 31.5 (High); Net carb= 43.7 g

Rice White—Cooked (cooked without added fat) ☛ Serving size= 1 cup, cooked (158 g); GI= 72 (High); GL= 31.4 (High); Net carb= 43.6 g

Rice White—Cooked Glutinous ☛ Serving size= 1 cup, cooked (174 g); GI= 86 (High); GL= 29.9 (High); Net carb= 34.7 g

Rice White—Glutinous Unenriched Cooked ☛ Serving size= 1 cup (174 g); GI= 86 (High); GL= 30.1 (High); Net carb= 35 g

Rice White—Glutinous Unenriched Uncooked ☛ Serving size= 1 cup (185 g); GI= 86 (High); GL= 125.5 (High); Net carb= 145.9 g

Rice White—Long-Grain Parboiled Unenriched Cooked ☛ Serving size= 1 cup (158 g); GI= 67 (Medium); GL= 26.6 (High); Net carb= 39.7 g

Rice White—Long-Grain Parboiled Unenriched Dry ☛ Serving size= 1 cup (185 g); GI= 67 (Medium); GL= 98 (High); Net carb= 146.3 g

Rice White—Long-Grain Parboiled, fortified Cooked ☛ Serving size= 1 cup (158 g); GI= 67 (Medium); GL= 26.6 (High); Net carb= 39.7 g

Rice White—Long-Grain Parboiled, fortified Dry ☛ Serving size= 1 cup (185 g); GI= 67 (Medium); GL= 98 (High); Net carb= 146.3 g

Rice White—Long-Grain Precooked Or Instant, fortified Dry ☛ Serving size= 1 cup (95 g); GI= 56 (Medium); GL= 42.8 (High); Net carb= 76.4 g

Rice White—Long-Grain Precooked Or Instant, fortified Prepared ☛ Serving size= 1 cup (165 g); GI= 56 (Medium); GL= 24.2 (High); Net carb= 43.2 g

Rice White—Long-Grain Raw ☛ Serving size= 1 cup (185 g); GI= 56 (Medium); GL= 81.5 (High); Net carb= 145.5 g

Rice White—Long-Grain Regular Cooked Unenriched With Salt ☛

Serving size= 1 cup (158 g); GI= 56 (Medium); GL= 24.6 (High); Net carb= 43.9 g

Rice White—Long-Grain Regular Cooked, fortified With Salt ☛ Serving size= 1 cup (158 g); GI= 56 (Medium); GL= 24.6 (High); Net carb= 43.9 g

Rice White—Long-Grain Regular Raw Unenriched ☛ Serving size= 1 cup (185 g); GI= 56 (Medium); GL= 81.5 (High); Net carb= 145.5 g

Rice White—Long-Grain Regular Unenriched Cooked Without Salt ☛ Serving size= 1 cup (158 g); GI= 56 (Medium); GL= 24.6 (High); Net carb= 43.9 g

Rice White—Medium-Grain Cooked Unenriched ☛ Serving size= 1 cup (186 g); GI= 65 (Medium); GL= 34.6 (High); Net carb= 53.2 g

Rice White—Medium-Grain Raw Unenriched ☛ Serving size= 1 cup (195 g); GI= 65 (Medium); GL= 100.6 (High); Net carb= 154.7 g

Rice White—Medium-Grain Raw, fortified ☛ Serving size= 1 cup (195 g); GI= 65 (Medium); GL= 98.8 (High); Net carb= 152 g

Rice White—Short-Grain Cooked Unenriched ☛ Serving size= 1 cup (205 g); GI= 72 (High); GL= 42.4 (High); Net carb= 58.9 g

Rice White—Short-Grain Raw Unenriched ☛ Serving size= 1 cup (200 g); GI= 72 (High); GL= 114 (High); Net carb= 158.3 g

Rice White—Short-Grain, fortified Cooked ☛ Serving size= 1 cup (186 g); GI= 72 (High); GL= 38.5 (High); Net carb= 53.4 g

Rice White—Short-Grain, fortified Uncooked ☛ Serving size= 1 cup (200 g); GI= 72 (High); GL= 109.9 (High); Net carb= 152.7 g

Rye Grain ☛ Serving size= 1 cup (169 g); GI= 59 (Medium); GL= 60.6 (High); Net carb= 102.7 g

Semolina Unenriched ☛ Serving size= 1 cup (167 g); GI= 66 (Medium); GL= 76 (High); Net carb= 115.1 g

Semolina, fortified ☛ Serving size= 1 cup (167 g); GI= 66 (Medium); GL= 76 (High); Net carb= 115.1 g

Sorghum Grain ☛ Serving size= 1 cup (192 g); GI= 66 (Medium); GL= 82.9 (High); Net carb= 125.5 g

Spaghetti made with whole wheat flour cooked ☛ Serving size= 2 oz (57 g); GI= 65 (Medium); GL= 22.1 (High); Net carb= 34 g

Spaghetti—100% durum wheat semolina cooked ☛ Serving size= 2 oz (57 g); GI= 58 (Medium); GL= 19.7 (High); Net carb= 34 g

Spaghetti—made with wheat flour cooked ☛ Serving size= 2 oz (57 g); GI= 60 (Medium); GL= 20.4 (High); Net carb= 34 g

Spaghetti—made with white wheat cooked ☛ Serving size= 2 oz (57 g); GI= 64 (Medium); GL= 21.8 (High); Net carb= 34 g

Spaghetti—Spinach Dry ☛ Serving size= 1 cup (140 g); GI= 33 (Low); GL= 29.7 (High); Net carb= 89.9 g

Spelt Uncooked ☛ Serving size= 1 cup (174 g); GI= 55 (Medium); GL= 56.9 (High); Net carb= 103.5 g

Tapioca Pearl Dry ☛ Serving size= 1 cup (152 g); GI= 70 (High); GL= 93.4 (High); Net carb= 133.4 g

Teff Uncooked ☛ Serving size= 1 cup (193 g); GI= 36 (Low); GL= 45.3 (High); Net carb= 125.7 g

Triticale ☛ Serving size= 1 cup (192 g); GI= 79 (High); GL= 109.4 (High); Net carb= 138.5 g

Triticale Flour Whole-Grain ☛ Serving size= 1 cup (130 g); GI= 79 (High); GL= 60.1 (High); Net carb= 76.1 g

Wheat Flour Whole-Grain ☛ Serving size= 1 cup (120 g); GI= 59 (Medium); GL= 43.4 (High); Net carb= 73.5 g

Wheat Flour Whole-Grain Soft Wheat ☛ Serving size= 1 cup (123 g); GI= 59 (Medium); GL= 44.5 (High); Net carb= 75.5 g

Wheat Germ Crude ☛ Serving size= 1 cup (115 g); GI= 59 (Medium); GL= 26.2 (High); Net carb= 44.4 g

Wheat Hard Red Spring ☛ Serving size= 1 cup (192 g); GI= 93 (High); GL= 99.7 (High); Net carb= 107.2 g

Wheat Hard Red Winter ☛ Serving size= 1 cup (192 g); GI= 93 (High); GL= 105.3 (High); Net carb= 113.2 g

Wheat Hard White ☛ Serving size= 1 cup (192 g); GI= 93 (High); GL= 113.7 (High); Net carb= 122.3 g

Wheat Kamut Khorasan Uncooked ☛ Serving size= 1 cup (186 g); GI= 40 (Low); GL= 44.3 (High); Net carb= 110.6 g

White Self-Rising Bolted Plain, fortified ☛ Serving size= 1 cup (122 g); GI= 68 (Medium); GL= 52.7 (High); Net carb= 77.6 g

Whole Grain Sorghum Flour ☛ Serving size= 1 cup (123 g); GI= 67 (Medium); GL= 57.7 (High); Net carb= 86.1 g

Wild Rice Raw ☛ Serving size= 1 cup (160 g); GI= 57 (Medium); GL= 62.7 (High); Net carb= 109.9 g

45

VEGETABLES

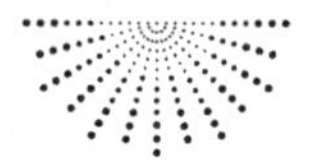

Cassava—cooked, without fat ☛ GI= 46 (Low); Serving size= 1 cup (206 g); GL= 34.1 (High); Net carb= 74.2 g

Corn Fritter ☛ GI= 65 (Medium); Serving size= 1 cup (107 g); GL= 26.9 (High); Net carb= 41.3 g

Corn Sweet White—Canned—Cream Style Regular Pack ☛ GI= 52 (Low); Serving size= 1 cup (256 g); GL= 23.2 (High); Net carb= 44.6 g

Corn Sweet Yellow—Canned—Cream Style Regular Pack ☛ GI= 52 (Low); Serving size= 1 cup (256 g); GL= 22.5 (High); Net carb= 43.3 g

Corn White—From Canned—Cream Style ☛ GI= 55 (Medium); Serving size= 1 cup (256 g); GL= 24.5 (High); Net carb= 44.5 g

Corn With Red And Green Peppers Canned—Solids And Liquids ☛ GI= 55 (Medium); Serving size= 1 cup (227 g); GL= 22.7 (High); Net carb= 41.2 g

Corn Yellow—From Canned—Cream Style ☛ GI= 62 (Medium); Serving size= 1 cup (256 g); GL= 26.8 (High); Net carb= 43.3 g

Corn Yellow—From Canned—Cream Style (cooked with fat) ☛ GI=

62 (Medium); Serving size= 1 cup (261 g); GL= 26.8 (High); Net carb= 43.3 g

Corn Yellow—Whole Kernel Frozen—Microwaved ☛ GI= 62 (Medium); Serving size= 1 cup (141 g); GL= 20.3 (High); Net carb= 32.8 g

Leeks (Bulb And Lower-Leaf Portion) Freeze-Dried ☛ GI= 32 (Low); Serving size= 1 cup (165 g); GL= 33.9 (High); Net carb= 106 g

Onion Rings Breaded Par Fried Frozen—Unprepared ☛ GI= 95 (High); Serving size= 6 rings (85 g); GL= 23.2 (High); Net carb= 24.4 g

Starchy Vegetables Including Tannier White Sweet Potato And Yam No Plantain ☛ GI= 84 (High); Serving size= 1 cup (190 g); GL= 48.8 (High); Net carb= 58.1 g

Starchy Vegetables Including Tannier White Sweet Potato And Yam With Green Or Ripe Plantains ☛ GI= 84 (High); Serving size= 1 cup (195 g); GL= 49.2 (High); Net carb= 58.6 g

Starchy Vegetables NFS Puerto Rican Style ☛ GI= 84 (High); Serving size= 1 cup (195 g); GL= 49.2 (High); Net carb= 58.6 g

Sweet Potato Canned—(cooked with fat) ☛ GI= 66 (Medium); Serving size= 1 cup, pieces (250 g); GL= 30.3 (High); Net carb= 45.9 g

Sweet Potato Canned—(cooked without fat) ☛ GI= 66 (Medium); Serving size= 1 cup, pieces (250 g); GL= 31.7 (High); Net carb= 48.1 g

Sweet Potato Casserole Or Mashed ☛ GI= 66 (Medium); Serving size= 1 cup (250 g); GL= 25.7 (High); Net carb= 39 g

White potato ☛ GI= 66 (Medium); Serving size= 1 medium (260 g); GL= 92.5 (High); Net carb= 15.8 g

White potato—baked, peel eaten, without fat ☛ GI= 73 (High); Serving size= 1 medium (260 g); GL= 127.9 (High); Net carb= 20 g

White potato—baked, peel not eaten ☛ GI= 73 (High); Serving size= 1 medium (260 g); GL= 121.7 (High); Net carb= 19 g

White potato—boiled, with peel, without fat ☛ GI= 66 (Medium); Serving size= 1 medium (260 g); GL= 96.7 (High); Net carb= 16.5 g

White potato—boiled, without peel, canned, low sodium, without fat ☛ GI= 63 (Medium); Serving size= 1 medium (260 g); GL= 91.4 (High); Net carb= 16.4 g

White potato—boiled, without peel, without fat ☛ GI= 66 (Medium); Serving size= 1 medium (260 g); GL= 94.7 (High); Net carb= 16.2 g

White potato—french fries, breaded or battered ☛ GI= 75 (High); Serving size= 1 medium (260 g); GL= 117.1 (High); Net carb= 17.7 g

White potato—french fries, from fresh, deep fried ☛ GI= 75 (High); Serving size= 1 medium (260 g); GL= 111 (High); Net carb= 16.7 g

White potato—french fries—From Frozen, deep fried ☛ GI= 75 (High); Serving size= 1 medium (260 g); GL= 125.1 (High); Net carb= 18.9 g

White potato—french fries—From Frozen, oven baked ☛ GI= 75 (High); Serving size= 1 medium (260 g); GL= 119.2 (High); Net carb= 18 g

White potato—from complete dry mix, mashed, made with water ☛ GI= 85 (High); Serving size= 1 medium (260 g); GL= 135.3 (High); Net carb= 18 g

White potato—from dry, mashed, made with milk, no fat ☛ GI= 85 (High); Serving size= 1 medium (260 g); GL= 135 (High); Net carb= 18 g

White potato—from fresh, mashed, made with milk ☛ GI= 79 (High); Serving size= 1 medium (260 g); GL= 126 (High); Net carb= 18 g

White potato—from fresh, mashed, not made with milk or fat ☛ GI= 79 (High); Serving size= 1 medium (260 g); GL= 133.5 (High); Net carb= 19.1 g

White potato—hash brown, from dry mix ☛ GI= 75 (High); Serving size= 1 medium (260 g); GL= 132.3 (High); Net carb= 20 g

White potato—hash brown, from fresh ☛ GI= 75 (High); Serving size= 1 medium (260 g); GL= 126.3 (High); Net carb= 19.1 g

White potato—hash brown—From Frozen ☛ GI= 75 (High); Serving size= 1 medium (260 g); GL= 126.6 (High); Net carb= 19.1 g

White potato—hash brown, with cheese ☛ GI= 75 (High); Serving size= 1 medium (260 g); GL= 126.3 (High); Net carb= 19.1 g

White potato—home fries ☛ GI= 75 (High); Serving size= 1 medium (260 g); GL= 126.3 (High); Net carb= 19.1 g

White potato—roasted, without fat ☛ GI= 73 (High); Serving size= 1 medium (260 g); GL= 122.1 (High); Net carb= 19.1 g

HEALTH AND NUTRITION WEBSITES

American Diabetes Association

(www.diabetes.org)

American Heart Association

(www.americanheart.org)

Centers for Disease Control and Prevention

(www.cdc.gov/healthyweight)

Cooking Light

(www.cookinglight.com)

Eating Well

(www.eatingwell.com)

eMedicine Health

(www.emedicinehealth.com)

Fruits and Vegetables Matter

(www.fruitsandveggiesmatter.gov)

Health

(www.health.com)

Hormone Foundation

(www.hormone.org)

National Heart, Lung, Blood Institute

(www.nhlbi.nih.gov)

National Institute on Aging

(www.nia.nih.gov)

National Institutes of Health

(http://health.nih.gov)

Nutrition.gov (www.nutrition.gov)

Prevention (www.prevention.com)